MEDICARE ESSENTIALS:

A PHYSICIAN INSIDER EXPLAINS THE FINE PRINT

Tanya Feke, MD

Cover Design by Createspace Cover Creator

ISBN-13: 978-0692218433 (Diagnosis Life. LLC)
ISBN-10: 0692218432

Dedications

Like you, I have faced challenges in my life and for that I am thankful. These challenges have shaped the woman I am today. The people I have met on this wild journey have made my life richer for the experience. It is to you that I am honored to have written this book.

Extra special love to my husband Gil and my children, Gilbert and Charlotte, who bring me joy every day. Your beautiful smiles fill my soul.

Special thanks to my family and friends who encourage me to follow my dreams. My writing could only happen with you at my side.

Special thanks to my patients over the years. It is because of you that I have become an advocate. Your stories have touched me in ways that have inspired me to be a better doctor and a better person.

To everyone, stay healthy!

MEDICARE ESSENTIALS: A Physician Insider Explains The Fine Print

Chapter 4 – Medicare and Prescriptions / Page 43

Chapter 5 – Medicare and Provider Visits / Page 73

Chapter 6 – Medicare and Outpatient Services / Page 91

Chapter 7 – Medicare in the Hospital / Page 121

Chapter 8 – Medicare in the Nursing Home and Beyond / Page 139

Chapter 9 – Medicare Checklists / Page 155

References / Page 175

Chapter 1 – Introduction

"We can never insure one-hundred percent of the population against one-hundred percent of the hazards and vicissitudes of life. But we have tried to frame a law which will give some measure of protection to the average citizen and to his family against the loss of a job and against poverty-ridden old age. This law, too, represents a cornerstone in a structure which is being built, but is by no means complete.... It is...a law that will take care of human needs and at the same time provide for the United States an economic structure of vastly greater soundness."

— Franklin D. Roosevelt

Meet Ms. Sandra Jones

Ms. Sandra Jones was born and raised in the United States. She had been married for 20 years but then divorced 10 years ago. She worked full time until this past month, when she retired. She kept the health benefits offered through her employer during that time. For this reason, she decided to defer applying for Medicare until "I really needed it." Now, she needed it. She signed up for Medicare on her sixty-eighth birthday. After all, it was free and she knew that all her medical expenses and medications would now be covered from here on out. Medicare takes care of all aspects of healthcare with one simple plan.

If you believe what Ms. Jones believes, you may be in trouble. Not everyone reads Medicare's fine print, especially not before they "need it". By then, it may be too late to prevent certain penalties from taking effect.

A simple overview of this government program can set realistic expectations for those who not only qualify for Medicare but also rely on it.

Who Am I?

"The buck stops here!"

— *Harry S. Truman*

I am the person you want on your side, the person smack-dab in the middle of it all. I am a family physician with years of clinical experience in the exam room and firsthand knowledge about insurers and that big old entity known as Medicare.

When I made the decision to become a doctor, my goal was to take care of people. After all, a physician cannot survive the grueling training in medical school and residency without that built-in altruism. The years of sacrifice are worth it to make a difference to the lives of the people in my community.

As it turns out, the field of medicine does not necessarily share that philosophy. This was the hardest lesson I learned as a practicing physician. There was always someone pushing me to see more patients, someone urging me to bill for more services, someone adding more administrative tasks to an overflowing list of responsibilities. What this did was leave me with less time to care for my patients. The essence of why I had become a doctor got muddied by the waters of big business.

Make no mistake: medicine is big business but not in the way you may think. It is not about corporate greed or sticking it to the American people. These are people's lives we are talking about. (No one will ever snuff that altruism out of me!) While the boards of for-profit hospitals may have a core objective of increasing the wealth of their investors, the U.S. medical system at large looks at things from a different perspective. The system aims to reduce costs so that resources can be better allocated for those people who need it. In the case of Medicare, that goal is to stretch those dollars out over as many years as possible before the bank goes bust. That is where healthcare reform comes in.

I do not fault any of my employers for trying to stay afloat during these challenging times, but medicine has evolved. My healthcare colleagues and I have been forced to adapt to more and more administrative red tape while caring for our patients on the front lines. Our patients do not understand why they are getting less time with their provider and in some cases getting billed more. We doctors are being looked upon as the bad guys while there are forces behind us that our patients may never appreciate.

This realization told me I needed to take a closer look at the forces pressuring our healthcare system. Where were the dollars coming from? Putting clinical practice aside, I dove into a career of utilization review and medical necessity compliance. While that may sound very technical, what it means is essentially this: I review real-life clinical cases and advise hospitals on whether they are appropriately utilizing, and billing for, their services. Instead of consulting with patients, I now consult with hospital networks.

The training required for my new role was extensive and many details are confidential by contract obligations. What I learned during this transition in my career, however, has been enlightening and even jaw-dropping. There is a whole other world behind that curtain with information I had never been privy to during my medical training. That was the point when I truly understood there was so much that people did not know about Medicare, doctors and patients alike. The trends I witnessed across my clinical career, and subsequently in my consulting career, need to be shared with the people who are affected most – Medicare beneficiaries.

I developed Diagnosis Life, a wellness web site at www.diagnosislife.com, to provide information to those of you trying to lead better, healthier lives. The site offers advice on common health ailments and gives you advice on how to live a more healthful life. It also takes some of the latest medical studies and cuts them down to size. Translating them from medical jargon to English is good for everyone. After all, some of the doctors I know have a hard time breaking down some of that information for themselves! The goal of the web site is to plant a seed that you have the power to make changes that will make you feel good about yourself inside and out.

Don't be too surprised by the movie content on my web site! Apart from being a family physician, I am also a film critic. One of the most important life lessons I have learned is that you need to find balance for your passions. For me those passions are medicine and film. Think of me as your movie doctor. I hope you can be inspired to do what makes you happy just the same.

A book seemed the next inevitable step on my journey to helping people make the most out of the current healthcare system. If you find this book helpful, I will have done my job. I hope you read on and encourage others to read this book as well.

What's In a Healthcare Provider?

I am a board certified family physician but I will not be the only provider you cross paths with as you make use of Medicare. There will be doctors of different specialties and graduates from medical schools both foreign and domestic who successfully trained in residency programs across the United States.

There will also be physician assistants (PA) and advanced practice nurse practitioners (APRN). While their training programs are different than that of a traditional physician, they are well versed in medicine and are mentored by physicians. In some states, physician supervision is not required. There remains some controversy in certain medical circles about whether or not physician supervision should be required, especially in areas where there is a shortage of doctors.

A PA or APRN may be your primary care provider in lieu of a physician. I make a point to mention this because I too often hear confusion about the roles of these alternate healthcare providers. I have had the good fortune to work with PAs and APRNs alike and have found many of them to be more knowledgeable than some physicians I have encountered. Simply stated, their expertise should not be belittled by their degree; to suggest otherwise is an insult to the profession. There are instances where Medicare requires a physician specifically to complete a given task. I will point out these situations to you as appropriate.

For the purposes of this book, I will frequently use the term provider to be inclusive to my healthcare colleagues. Together we provide care to millions of Americans. Together we need to adapt to the changes in Medicare.

Why You Need This Book

If you are reading this book, you are likely a Medicare recipient or at the very least you know someone who is. According to the Centers for Medicare and Medicaid Services (CMS), there were 50.8 million people on Medicare in 2012. When looking at data from the United States Census Bureau, that was 16% of the population.

FACT CHECK:

In 2012, 50.8 million Americans were covered by Medicare.

With an increasing number of baby boomers reaching Medicare eligibility age, the number of people enrolled in Medicare is expected to jump to 57 million by 2020. Add to that the fact that our estimated life expectancy is on the rise. CMS reports that a man aged 65 years old in 2020 will be expected to live an additional 18.8 years, a woman 21.1 years. While that may be good news for us as individuals, the United States government may not be quite ready to pop a cork on that bottle of champagne. With Medicare accountable to nearly sixty million beneficiaries over several decades, at the very least, will there be enough money to pull it off?

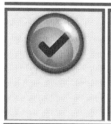

FACT CHECK:

For 2020, life expectancies are projected to increase to 83.8 years for men and 86.1 years for women.

To accommodate an aging population, Medicare has and will continue to make changes over the years to not only improve efficiency but also to contain costs. Some of these changes will benefit the population at large. Reducing Medicare fraud, for example, will allow more funds to be freed up for everyone. But not all changes will be met with open arms.

Everyone wants to know: What is the cost to ME?

It does not feel good when change affects you on a personal level. Medicare is sure to affect you whether you or a loved one relies on its services. The unfortunate truth is that many misconceptions exist about what Medicare does and does not provide, what it covers and what it does not cover. Too much is buried in the fine print.

FINE PRINT:

These boxes will be displayed throughout the book to summarize key details often misunderstood or buried in the "fine print".

The purpose of this book is not to spell out every minutia about Medicare. You can always go to government-owned web sites like www.medicare.gov and www.cms.gov for that. The goal is to show you the most common features of Medicare that stump beneficiaries, how they are often misunderstood and how understanding where the money goes can put some back into your own pockets. A rare Medicare guide written by a physician, this book also shows you how to get better clinical care.

Chapter 2 - Medicare Essentials

*"One of the most urgent orders of business at this time is the
enactment of hospital insurance for the aged through Social
Security to help older people meet the high costs of illness without
jeopardizing their economic independence."*

— *Lyndon B. Johnson*

Medicare in a Nutshell

Simply put, Medicare is government sponsored healthcare that came into law as part of the Social Security Act of 1965. Initially intended to provide services for those on Social Security, it has evolved to become the main source of healthcare coverage for the majority of people aged 65 years of age and older in this country. It acts like private insurance. From that endorsement alone, it should be easy to see that Medicare is not free. Like an insurance company, there are out-of-pocket expenses that you, the beneficiary, will be expected to pay.

Medicare Eligibility

To be eligible for Medicare, a person must first be a United States citizen or a permanent legal resident. Legal residency must be established over 5 years. Citizens and legal residents older than 65 years old are eligible for Medicare. Further, individuals with certain medical disabilities may be eligible regardless of age.

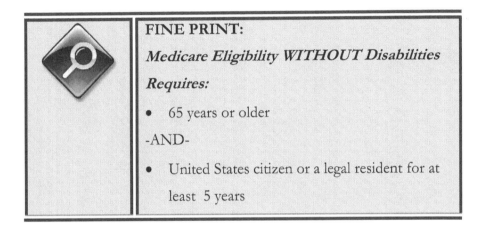

FINE PRINT:

Medicare Eligibility WITHOUT Disabilities Requires:

- 65 years or older

-AND-

- United States citizen or a legal resident for at least 5 years

Working in Medicare-eligible employment is not a formal requirement for Medicare coverage. Medicare-eligible employment simply means that the Medicare applicant or his/her spouse paid Medicare taxes to the government over a defined period of time. These payroll taxes do play a major role in how much someone will pay for Medicare coverage when they become eligible for care by the criteria outlined here. Medicare-eligible employment will be discussed further in Chapter 3.

An individual who has permanent kidney failure, also known as end stage renal disease (ESRD), is eligible for Medicare at any age if he or she needs dialysis or is in need of or has had a kidney transplant, though that alone is not enough to get onto Medicare's roster.

The A, B, C, D of Medicare

Medicare services are divided across four categories – A, B, C and D. Medicare Parts A and B are often called "classic" Medicare as they cover the "nuts and bolts" of healthcare needs. Medicare Parts C and D are optional and require additional expenditures by the enrollee.

Medicare Part A covers hospital and emergency care. These services can extend beyond hospital walls to include rehabilitation facilities, nursing homes, hospice and home healthcare offerings. Nothing is ever black and white: certain criteria must be met in order for Medicare to pay for these services.

Medicare Part B covers outpatient care such as doctor's visits, ambulance services, routine tests, diabetic supplies and preventive services. Preventive services are intended to prevent disease from occurring in the first place or to identify diseases in their earlier stages to allow for more effective treatment early on. Services provided in Part B must be considered medically necessary. We will get back to that in a later chapter.

Medicare Part C is known as the Medicare Advantage Plan. These optional plans allow enrollees to purchase healthcare coverage from private insurance companies approved by Medicare. Depending on the Medicare Advantage Plan selected, costs will vary with different copays and deductibles. Some of these plans may be more cost effective for certain individuals as they combine Part A, Part B and sometimes Part D coverage into one plan.

Medicare Part D covers outpatient prescription medications and, similarly to Part C, is offered through private insurance companies approved by Medicare. Part D was added in 2003. Selection is made based on a person's needs from the many plans available. Each plan has different associated costs depending on how narrow or broad the drug coverage is. It is important to note that medications used during a hospital stay are covered under Part A.

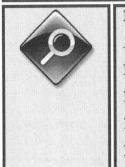

FINE PRINT:

Medicare Parts Overview

Part A: Hospital coverage (INPATIENT)

Part B: Medical coverage (OUTPATIENT)

Part C: Medicare Advantage Plans

Part D: Prescription coverage

The Affordable Care Act and Medicare

If there is one thing that has been said time and again by the Obama administration, it is that Medicare will not be affected by the Affordable Care Act (ACA). Changes to the healthcare market place do not change someone's eligibility or access to Medicare. The care access you have today will not be any different than what you had before Congress approved the ACA, widely known as Obamacare, in 2010. However, this is not entirely true.

Supporters of the law claim that Medicare will actually strengthen under the new health law. Since Medicare is not part of the health insurance marketplace set forth by the ACA, its coverage to beneficiaries will not be directly changed. However, changes have taken place since the ACA has passed that have impacted Medicare.

For one, prescription drug coverage has improved for brand name medications.

THE PROBLEM:

This only happens after you have spent a certain amount and only decreases costs by 50% from market prices for a limited period of time.

When you think about it, it means that you have to spend more money to save ANY money. Are we encouraging seniors towards using more brand name products? What is the donut hole? These and other issues will be addressed in Chapter 4.

Medicare coverage has expanded to include preventive services such as wellness visits and screening tests such as mammograms and colonoscopies—for free! After all, an ounce of prevention is worth a pound of cure.

THE PROBLEM:

The government and many healthcare providers do not always agree on what preventive services should be offered.

It all comes down to medical necessity. These magic words have become the focus of all of healthcare. Understanding how to make the most out of these services will be the focus of Chapter 5.

The impact that the ACA has on Medicare involves cost shifting. Uncovering Medicare fraud could save millions of dollars for the Medicare Trust Fund. This, in addition to streamlining certain efficiencies in Medicare, is expected to preserve Medicare for future generations. Before 2010, Medicare funds were expected to last through 2017; the ACA extends this to at least 2029.

Ms. Jones Signs Up For Medicare

Ms. Jones had many misconceptions about Medicare. It was not as simple or straightforward as she thought. Depending on where and how she received her healthcare, she would rely on different aspects of the program.

One day she took a sudden fall in the snow and fractured her hip. This required a hospital stay and hip surgery. Medicare Part A would cover the hospital expenses after she paid a deductible. It would also cover her medication costs during the time of the hospitalization.

She was later discharged from the hospital and returned home. At that point, Medicare Part A coverage would no longer be in effect. When she saw her doctor for a follow-up visit, her costs would be covered by Medicare Part B. Again, she would be expected to pay a percentage of the fees. Any medications the doctor prescribed would be covered by Medicare Part D after copays, if she had selected one of the Part D plans.

If she had a Medicare Advantage Plan, it is possible her Medicare costs would have all defaulted to Medicare Part C, depending on the specific plan she selected.

Not so clear cut is it? Specific costs associated with Medicare will be addressed next.

Chapter 3 – Direct Costs of Medicare

"In this world nothing can be said to be certain, except death and taxes".

— *Benjamin Franklin*

Medicare Taxes

Most people have paid well in advance for Medicare. Years of taxes have contributed to the federal government's funding for the program. Those dollars are taken paycheck after paycheck with the promise that Medicare will provide coverage to that individual once he or she reaches eligibility age. How long, rather than how much, one pays into the system decides how much he or she will have to pay out of pocket when starting to use Medicare.

Monthly Premiums

Another cost expenditure that many do not consider until they are in the throes of Medicare is the monthly premium. Part A coverage may be free for certain beneficiaries but Parts B, C and D each have a separate cost.

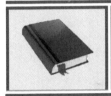

DEFINITION:

A <u>premium</u> is a fee paid periodically, such as every month, for a service.

The cost of Part A coverage is waived for those meeting the disability criteria discussed previously. The monthly premiums will also be waived for eligible applicants 65 years of age and older who meet residency requirements and who have contributed Medicare payroll taxes for at least 10 years. If an individual has not contributed to Medicare payroll taxes personally, that individual is equally eligible if his/her spouse or former spouse had done so.

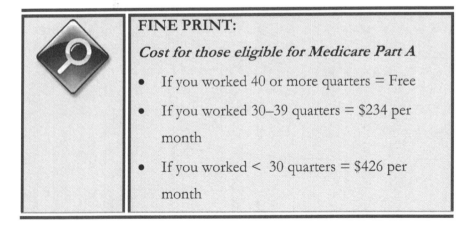

FINE PRINT:

Cost for those eligible for Medicare Part A

- If you worked 40 or more quarters = Free
- If you worked 30–39 quarters = $234 per month
- If you worked < 30 quarters = $426 per month

The government looks at tax contributions in terms of quarters. Forty calendar quarters (10 years) are required to receive Part A coverage for free. An individual who has contributed less needs to pay a monthly premium for Part A services that depends on how many quarters he/she did pay Medicare taxes. For those who contributed between 30 and 39 quarters of taxes, their monthly premium in 2014 will be $234.00. For those who contributed less than 30 quarters, their monthly premium will be $426.00.

In 2014, Part B costs range from $104.90 per month to $335.70 per month depending on an individual's prior tax returns. The lower-end premiums apply to those earning less than $85,000 on their individual tax returns or less than $170,000 on a joint tax return. The upper-end premiums target those earning more than $214,000 (individual) or $428,000 (joint). Medicare uses tax returns from 2 years prior to eligibility to determine how much you should pay for your premium. There is also a deductible of $147 per year to consider. All of these costs may be adjusted on an annual basis.

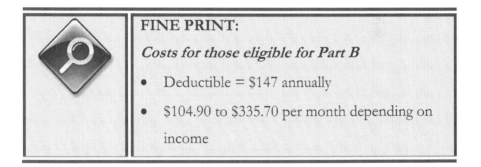

FINE PRINT:

Costs for those eligible for Part B

- Deductible = $147 annually
- $104.90 to $335.70 per month depending on income

Premiums for Part C and Part D have greater variability as these parts of Medicare are run by private insurance companies. While Part D premiums differ depending on the specific policy you choose, the lowest cost will be $32.42. This is known as the national base beneficiary premium and the dollar amount changes every year. However, additional costs may be tagged onto the monthly premium.

For those earning less than $85,000 on their individual tax returns or less than $170,000 on a joint tax return, there is no added cost. For those with higher incomes, an extra $12.30 to $69.30 is added to the premium cost every month. These costs reflect the rates for 2014.

Similar to Part B, income tax returns from 2 years prior are used to decide how much you will pay.

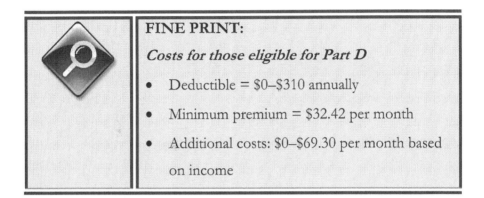

FINE PRINT:

Costs for those eligible for Part D

- Deductible = $0–$310 annually

- Minimum premium = $32.42 per month

- Additional costs: $0–$69.30 per month based on income

Late Fees

Late fees are applied to those who sign up for Part A, Part B and/or Part D after initial eligibility deadlines. This is where a little knowledge goes a long way. The enrollment window is actually quite narrow: it begins 3 months before your 65th birthday and extends 3 months after that birthday. People who have existing health insurance through their employer or their spouse's employer may have additional special enrollment options once that coverage runs out without having to pay Medicare penalties when they finally do sign up.

FINE PRINT:

Eligibility Period = +/- 3 months from your 65th birthday

Medicare's late penalties are based on how long a person could have had coverage. Part A adds 10% to the monthly premiums for twice the number of years a person had been eligible before they signed up. A year is defined as a full 12 month period. For example, if someone was eligible for Part A two years before they signed up, they will pay the higher premium for four years (twice the number of years) before they can return to the original premium rate.

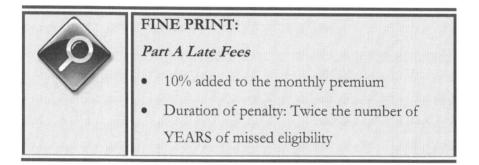

FINE PRINT:

Part A Late Fees

- 10% added to the monthly premium
- Duration of penalty: Twice the number of YEARS of missed eligibility

FINE PRINT:

Part B Late Fees

- 10% added to the monthly premium for every YEAR of missed eligibility
- Duration of penalty: Long-standing

Part B, similarly tags on an extra 10% to premiums but does so for every year that a person had been eligible for Part B. For example, if someone was eligible for Part B two years before they signed up, they will pay 20% (number of years times 10%) more in premiums each month. The added costs go on indefinitely and do not end like the penalties in Part A.

A 1% late enrollment Part D penalty will be added for every month you were eligible and did not have prescription drug coverage from another source. This Part D late fee is calculated off of the national base beneficiary premium of $32.42 rather than the higher premiums from the different plans some people will choose. Since the national base beneficiary premium can change from year to year, the late penalty will change as well but you will pay the penalty for the life of your coverage. Yes, you will be penalized as long as you have Medicare Part D. The one exception to this penalty occurs if your eligibility began before the age of 65. Once you turn 65 years old, the penalty will be removed.

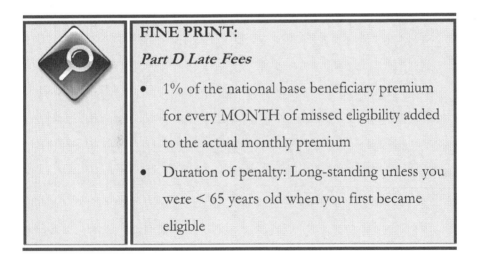

FINE PRINT:

Part D Late Fees

- 1% of the national base beneficiary premium for every MONTH of missed eligibility added to the actual monthly premium
- Duration of penalty: Long-standing unless you were < 65 years old when you first became eligible

Altogether, these Medicare costs quickly add up and beneficiaries require thoughtful preparation before they jump into the fray. They need to do their research on what plans will work best for them, and in a timely manner to avoid costly penalties.

Deductibles, Coinsurance and Copays

Paying monthly premiums does not mean that the rest of your healthcare is provided free of charge. Deductibles, coinsurance and copays factor strongly into the equation.

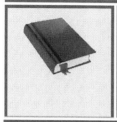

DEFINITION:

A <u>deductible</u> is a fixed dollar amount you pay for healthcare services before your insurance coverage kicks in.

Part A deductibles are costly. For each inpatient hospital stay up to 60 days in 2014, there is a deductible of $1,216. That means you will pay the same amount whether you stay 2 days or 60 days. Not that anyone wants to be in the hospital longer, but in one sense, the longer you stay the bigger the bargain. On the other hand, costs begin to accrue for stays longer than that. For day 61 to 90, there is an added price tag of $304 per day and for stays after 91 days, a cost of $608 dollars per day. For stays 91 days and longer, you start to dig into your lifetime reserve days. Medicare allows only for coverage of a maximum 60 reserve days in your lifetime.* After that, you will pay full out-of-pocket expenses.

The billing cycle starts all over again if you are discharged from the hospital and are admitted to the hospital another time. As an example, if you are admitted to the hospital in January, you will pay the $1,216 deductible and costs for added days as noted above. If you stay 92 days total, you will have used up two of your lifetime reserve days, leaving you with 58 days. If you are admitted to the hospital again in

June, you will pay another $1,216 deductible and so on. For your health and wellbeing, I pray you do not require repeated hospital stays that long.

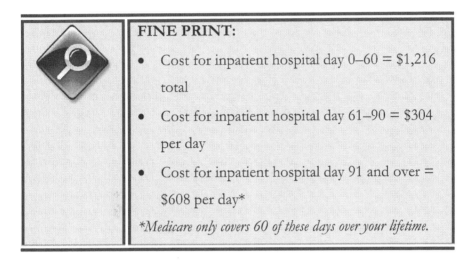

FINE PRINT:

- Cost for inpatient hospital day 0–60 = $1,216 total
- Cost for inpatient hospital day 61–90 = $304 per day
- Cost for inpatient hospital day 91 and over = $608 per day*

Medicare only covers 60 of these days over your lifetime.

Costs are calculated differently for stays in a skilled nursing facility. Examples of skilled nursing facilities are rehabilitation centers and nursing homes as long as they provide certain levels of care. The details will be discussed in Chapter 8. There is no deductible for stays in a skilled nursing facility up to 20 days for each eligible admission. For days 21 to 100, however, you will be charged $152 per day as coinsurance. After that time, you will be responsible for all costs. Lifetime reserve days do not apply.

Part D deductibles will vary based on the prescription plan you choose. Some may have no deductible while the maximum deductible allowable is $310 for 2014. This capped amount changes on an annual basis.

DEFINITION:

A <u>coinsurance</u> is a fixed percentage you pay for a product or service. The cost you pay will differ depending on how expensive the item is.

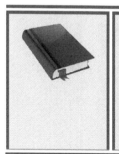

DEFINITION:

A <u>copayment</u> or <u>copay</u> is a fixed fee you pay every time you purchase a product or service. Regardless of the cost of the item, your payment will always be the same.

Part B requires that you pay a coinsurance with the exception of Wellness visits and specific preventive medicine services which are free. These coinsurance costs, often 20%, apply to outpatient services ranging from doctor's appointments to laboratory tests to diabetic supplies. This will be addressed in detail in Chapter 4.

Part D services usually require a copay or coinsurance for purchases of medication. This will also be addressed in Chapter 4.

Cost Summaries

The expected costs for 2014, including potential late fees, are broken down in the following tables for Parts A, B and D.

Medicare Part A: Expected Costs in 2014
Based on Quarters of Medicare Eligible Employment

	40+ quarters	30–39 quarters	< 30 quarters
Monthly premium	$0	$234	$426
Late penalty	$0	$23.40	$42.60
Monthly premium with penalty	$0	$257.40	$468.60
Annual cost	$0	$2,808	$5,112
Annual cost with penalty	$0	$3,088.80	$5,623.20

Medicare Part B: Expected Costs in 2014
Based on Income Tax Returns

	Single: < $85,000 -or- Joint: < $170,000 Married/Separate: < $85,000	Single: $85,000–$107,00 -or- Joint: $170,000–$214,000 Married/Separate: N/A	Single : $107,000–$160,000 –or- Joint: $214,000–$320,000 Married/Separate: N/A	Single: $160,000–$214,000 -or- Joint: $320,000–$428,000 Married/Separate: $85,000–$129,000	Single: > $214,000 -or- Joint: > $428,000 Married/Separate: > $129,000
Monthly Premium	$104.90	$146.90	$209.80	$272.70	$335.70
Deductible	$147	$147	$147	$147	$147
Annual Cost	$1,259	$1,763	$2,518	$3,264	$4028
A late penalty of 10% is added to the monthly premium for every YEAR of missed enrollment after eligibility, i.e. one year = 10%, two years = 20%, three years = 30% etc.					

Medicare Part D: Expected Costs in 2014
Based on Quarters of Medicare Eligible Employment

	Single: < $85,000 -or- Joint: < $170,000 Married/Separate: < $85,000	Single: $85,000–$107,00 -or- Joint: $170,000–$214,000 Married/Separate: N/A	Single : $107,000–$160,000 -or- Joint: $214,000–$320,000 Married/Separate: N/A	Single: $160,000–$214,000 -or- Joint: $320,000–$428,000 Married/Separate: $85,000 - $129,000	Single: > $214,000 -or- Joint: > $428,000 Married/Separate: > $129,000
Monthly Premium	Variable ($32.42 min)				
Added Costs	$0	$12.10	$31.10	$50.20	$69.30
Deductible	$0–$310				
Annual Cost (Min)	$389	$534	$762	$991	$1,220

A late penalty of 1% of the national base beneficiary premium ($32.42 in 2014) rounded to the nearest $0.10 is added to the monthly premium for every full MONTH of missed enrollment after eligibility, i.e. 10 months = $3.20, 20 months = $6.50, 30 months = $9.70 etc.

Medicare Assignment

All this discussion about costs has been getting a little expensive, wouldn't you say? It can get a whole lot more pricey depending on what healthcare provider you choose. There are two important things that you need to ask your provider before you get started.

The first thing to know is obvious and instinctive: does your provider take Medicare patients? If your provider has opted out of Medicare, he can charge you whatever he wants and you will be responsible for those costs out of your own pocket. Medicare will not pay even for services usually covered by Medicare.

In this case, that provider may ask that you sign a private contract to review the finer details of your financial obligations. This contract, however, cannot include a clause for urgent or emergency care—it would not be ethical for a provider to turn you away because of dollars and cents in times of a true emergency.

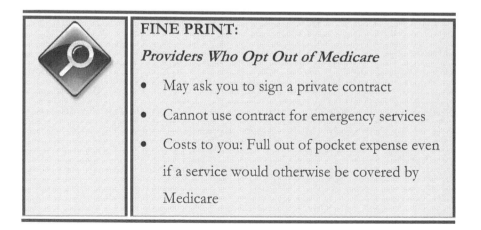

FINE PRINT:

Providers Who Opt Out of Medicare

- May ask you to sign a private contract

- Cannot use contract for emergency services

- Costs to you: Full out of pocket expense even if a service would otherwise be covered by Medicare

It is in your best interest, financially at least, to seek out healthcare providers who do accept Medicare. At times you may not have a choice if there are limited resources in your area capable of providing proper care.

For those providers who do opt in for Medicare there is another important distinction: does the provider accept assignment or not? Medicare sets a fee schedule for all covered services. Accepting assignment means that your provider has signed a contract with the government agreeing to all of these fixed fees. Furthermore, they will only charge you the amount of your coinsurance and Medicare deductible, not more. This fee schedule keeps the costs to you as low as possible regardless of where you live in the country.

FINE PRINT:

Participating Provider

Accepts Medicare fee schedule in full

Costs to you: Coinsurance + deductible

Non-participating providers who do accept Medicare as insurance may accept only some of the set fees or none at all. They can charge you up to 15% more than the cost recommended by Medicare. This "limiting charge" is an attempt at cost containment so that no more than 15% of the cost will be added on top of your usual coinsurance and deductible. Unfortunately, limiting charges do not apply to durable medical equipment and non-participating suppliers of that equipment. These suppliers can charge you whatever they want. A list of durable medical equipment is provided in Chapter 4.

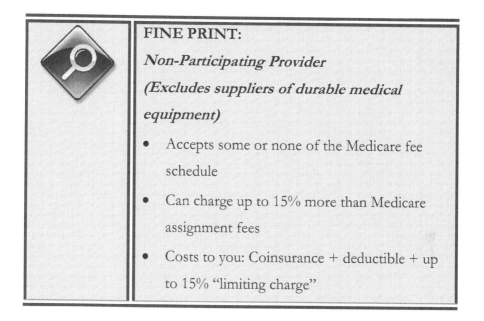

FINE PRINT:

Non-Participating Provider

(Excludes suppliers of durable medical equipment)

- Accepts some or none of the Medicare fee schedule
- Can charge up to 15% more than Medicare assignment fees
- Costs to you: Coinsurance + deductible + up to 15% "limiting charge"

Unless otherwise stated, the costs described later in this book will refer to those of participating providers accepting assignment.

ICD Codes

It should not be surprising that medical billing is not a straightforward and simple process. Your healthcare provider cannot simply write down hypertension and generate a bill for services. Every diagnosis is associated with its own code and your provider has to choose the right one. That is not always as easy as it sounds.

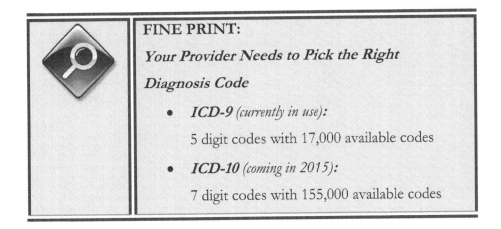

FINE PRINT:

Your Provider Needs to Pick the Right Diagnosis Code

- *ICD-9 (currently in use):*
  5 digit codes with 17,000 available codes

- *ICD-10 (coming in 2015):*
  7 digit codes with 155,000 available codes

The International Classification of Diseases (ICD) is a system of codes used to monitor diagnoses worldwide. The World Health Organization heads revisions to ICD every 10 years. The ICD system currently used in the United States, ICD-9, has more than 17,000 codes available. ICD-9 codes may be up to 5 digits long. There are many different diagnoses for the same type of problem. For example, the specific hypertension code will depend on what is causing the hypertension and whether there is also associated heart or kidney disease among other factors. Medicare and other insurers may recognize certain codes as acceptable while denying others for payment. That puts a lot of pressure on your healthcare provider.

ICD-10 is already here and being used in other countries. The United States has been slow to implement it and with good reason. It is a drastic change, expanding to 7 digits and more than 155,000 different codes. The government has delayed implementation of ICD-10 use for two years in a row now. The American Medical Association has had a strong voice in lobbying against the transition, which explains to some extent the repeated delays. The next expected implementation date for ICD-10 is set for October 2015. If your provider is having trouble now, it is not going to get easier. There may be a rocky transition.

If you feel you have received a charge or bill in error, it could be due to a coding problem. Your healthcare provider may need to change a diagnostic code for services to be covered by Medicare. You may need to contact your provider's medical or billing office to address the issue.

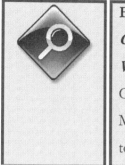

FINE PRINT:

Overcharging May be Due to Using the Wrong Diagnosis Code

Contact your healthcare provider to see if Medicare requires another diagnosis code in order to pay for services rendered.

Ms. Jones Spends a Fortune

Looking back to Ms. Jones, it is easy to see now that her assumptions about Medicare were incorrect. At sixty eight years old, she is three years past her eligibility date. The late penalties could automatically kick in. Thankfully, she had health insurance under her employer in the meantime and could apply during a special enrollment period. Otherwise, she would have had to increase her Part A monthly premium by 10% for six years.

Her Part B premium will automatically be increased by 30% per month which could be an extra $30 to $100 per month or $360 to $1200 per year. This penalty will last as long as she has Medicare. For someone on a fixed income, this could mean the difference between affording rent, food or prescription medications.

The hospital stay for her hip fracture also tagged on a Part A deductible cost of $1,216 and her outpatient follow-up visit medications required she pay 20% of the visit expenses from Part B in addition to any medication copays for Part D.

Maybe Medicare was not as inexpensive as she thought.

Chapter 4 - Medicare At Home

A hip fracture was not the only health problem that Ms. Jones faced. She also has a history for diabetes for which she takes oral medications. She needs refills on her medications and she also needs supplies to monitor her sugar levels. She looks to Medicare to cover these expenses but can she find the best deal?

People use Medicare to help pay for many of their day to day expenses. Prescription medications and medical supplies are big business. According to the IMS Institute for Healthcare Informatics, prescription medications cost the nation $325.8 billion in 2012 with the average person spending $898 out of pocket to pay for them. Understanding when and where you can cut costs can make a difference not only for those on Medicare but for all healthcare consumers.

Prescriptions by the Numbers

"The doctor of the future will give no medicine, but will interest his patient in the care of the human frame, in diet and in the cause and prevention of disease."

— Thomas Jefferson

I would like to think of myself as a doctor of the future. Like Thomas Jefferson, I promote healthy lifestyle choices before looking to medications. Eat healthy. Exercise regularly. Stay positive. The unfortunate truth is that medications are sometimes necessary to treat a condition or to at least minimize symptoms. On graduation day from medical school, I took an oath to alleviate pain and suffering.

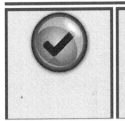

FACT CHECK:

In 2011, the United States Census Bureau reported the average person over 65 years old filled 28.5 prescriptions.

If you are one of the lucky ones, your dependence on prescription medications will be minimal as you age. The statistics unfortunately are stacked against you. According to the United States Census Bureau, the average person over 65 years old filled 28.5 prescriptions in 2011. This number does not mean that a person received 28.5 different medications from their pharmacy. This number includes refills for the same medication.

With that in mind, one medication could represent anywhere from 1 to 12 prescriptions depending on how many refills that medication required. Most prescriptions are filled in 30 day or 90 day supplies so a more reflective estimate would be to say that the average person over 65 years old takes 2 to 7 different prescription medications per year.

A separate survey looking at both prescription and over the counter medications was reported in the Journal of the American Medical Association in 2008. Of 3005 adults between the ages of 57 and 85 years old, 81% used at least one medication and 29% used five or more medications. For those older than 75 years old, five or more medications were used by as many as 36% of those surveyed. The point is that there are a lot of medications being prescribed on a regular basis and therefore opportunities for saving.

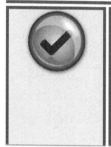

FACT CHECK:

In 2008, a survey in the Journal of the American Medical Association estimated that 36% of people over 75 years old used five or more medications (prescription and over-the-counter).

Medication Price Tag

Some generic medications cost cents on the dollar while others cost thousands of dollars for one dose. Examples can be seen in the brand name products HUMIRA®[1] and ENBREL®[2] used to treat

---

[1] HUMIRA is a registered trademark of is a registered trademark of AbbVie.

complicated diseases such as rheumatoid arthritis and psoriasis. Without insurance, these medications may cost up to $2,700 to $2,900, respectively, for a one month supply. One could easily go bankrupt paying these costs out-of-pocket but if these medications could mean the difference between quality living and suffering, what would your health be worth?

Enter insurance. Insurance allows a person to pay a small portion of the expense, a copay, while their insurance pays the difference. Often the insurance company has negotiated a price with the pharmaceutical company for certain medications. This is how formularies come into play. Formularies are essentially a preferred list of medications for you to choose from.

Different insurance companies will have different formularies. The intention is to save both you and your insurance money, but to be honest, more for your insurance. If a medication is not on your formulary, your health insurance may require you to go through a special approval process to get the medication or they can deny coverage altogether, shifting the entire cost to you. It is in your best interest to have your healthcare provider prescribe medications from your formulary to help keep costs down.

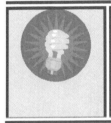

CONCEPT:

Insurance companies negotiate the prices of medications with pharmaceutical companies and pharmacies to save money.

---

[2] ENBREL is a registered trademark of Amgen.

People tend to think of insurance companies as the "bad guy" but, after all, they are in business and an insurance company wants to cut costs as much as you do. By encouraging you to pick medications that they get a bargain on, the insurance companies pay less of a cost differential than with other medications. By getting you to pick the least expensive medications, they save even more.

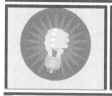

CONCEPT:

Total medication cost − your copay = What Medicare Part D pays

Medications are ranked using a tier system according to your insurance plan, Medicare Part D or otherwise. Generic drugs are often on tier 1 while tiers 2 and above may offer more expensive brand name products. The higher the tier, the higher the copay.

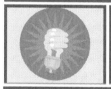

CONCEPT:

The higher the tier, the higher the copay.

You will pay a copay each time you fill a prescription whether it is a medication new to you or not. Copays can range from a few dollars up to $30 for each prescription. Considering the average adult over 65 years old pays for 28.5 copays per year, that could quickly add up to a lot of money.

Brand Name vs. Generic Debate

It fascinates me how loyal some people are to brand name products. If someone has stock in a company, that is one thing. The majority of the time, however, the preference for a brand name is for the purpose of some presumed status or reputation. People like belonging to a prestigious group. They like having the best of the best.

Let me fill you in on a little secret: brand-name loyalty in medicine is not necessary. It rarely matters. A generic version of a branded medication is by definition the same chemical compound as its counterpart. With the same ingredient and the same dose strength, the clinical effect should technically be the same.

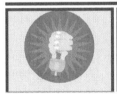

CONCEPT:

Generic medications are often as good as brand name medications.

Like anything in life, however, there are shades of gray. There may be times when a medication is processed differently between pharmaceutical companies. Perhaps the mechanism for deriving or purifying the drug is unique at one facility versus another, even though the final product—the active ingredient—is the same.

With this in mind, there remains a possibility that a person may react differently to one generic medication versus another generic or the branded product. For example, residue of a processing chemical could be present on the drug. Some of my patients have developed an allergic reaction to a generic version of a medication while tolerating the brand-name version. I have seen it go so far as a patient responding well to a generic medication from one pharmaceutical company but not the same generic medication from another company. The reverse effect is also possible: an individual tolerating a generic version of a drug over the brand name. Of course some sort of placebo effect could be at play here too, but these examples illustrate rare occasions when a brand-name product may be indicated. Again, this is the exception rather than the rule.

Not all medications have a generic version on the market. A medication may still be under patent by the pharmaceutical company that discovered that drug. In this scenario, generic versions of the medication cannot be made by other companies until that patent expires. Once the patent runs out, generic medications may be made by one and often several other companies which decreases costs of the medication by virtue of competition. Good old capitalism at work.

A medication could also be the first of its kind or in a class that only has brand-name medications available. HUMIRA and ENBREL are perfect examples of this sort of medication, which explains, to some extent, their high cost. If other classes of medications are not effective or appropriate for an individual, a healthcare provider may need to prescribe one of these more costly medications.

The lesson to learn here is simple: sometimes brand-name medications are necessary and sometimes they are not.

Switching from Brand-Name to Generic

Insurance companies will often send requests to their beneficiaries suggesting changes from a brand-name to a generic medication. Healthcare providers receive similar mailings. The intention is to cut costs for both the beneficiary and the insurance company. You may have a lower copay and your insurance will pay less when they pay the cost difference for a cheaper medication.

Before you pounce on the offer, be sure that there is actually a generic version of the medication available. Oftentimes insurance companies will include generic medications on that mailing list that are in the same class of medications but are not actually the same drug.

FINE PRINT:

Switching to a generic medication with the same active ingredient will likely have the same effect on your body.

This is where the insurance companies begin to think more about their bottom line than what may be best for your health. It is not ill will that they do this. Often medications in the same class, meaning that they work by the same mechanism of action, have the same or a similar effect on an individual. This cannot be guaranteed, however.

Everyone has a different metabolism and may respond differently to another medication, even if it works in the same way. If a medication has had a positive clinical effect on a person, it seems a shame to change it unnecessarily. A generic of the same exact medication, however, is a very reasonable option.

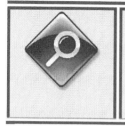

FINE PRINT:

Switching to a generic medication in the same class of medication may or may not have the same effect on your body.

Let us use an example I came across hundreds of times in my career. Ms. Jones had been taking Lexapro®[3], a medication for depression. It is a brand name product in the family of selective serotonin receptor inhibitors (SSRIs). Before it went generic, insurance companies would send letters to my patients asking them to replace the medication with a generic option. Many of my patients took this to mean there was a generic version of Lexapro when there was not. There were, however, many generic SSRI options available. An important fact to know about SSRIs is that their clinical effect may not "kick in" for several weeks.

- Will another medication in the class have the same effect as Lexapro?
- If Lexapro had been working well for her, is it worth risking a worsening of her depression while trying another medicine?
- Are the cost savings worth it?

The answer will vary for each person. Your personal value system will come into play. As a physician, the health of my patient comes first and foremost.

---

[3] Lexapro is a registered trademark of Forest Pharmaceuticals, Inc.

The scenario above could be the case for any brand-name medication. This is not a marketing campaign for Lexapro, only a common example I encountered in my clinical practice and as I mentioned, generic versions of medication are now available.

As a doctor, my brand name loyalty to drug companies is a big fat nil. Which leads me to free samples…

The Good and Bad of Free Samples

Many doctor's offices provide free medication samples while others are steering away from this practice. Traditionally, pharmaceutical companies send representatives to visit with medical offices to deliver the samples while also promoting their products. These representatives may provide literature and studies reporting benefits of the medication while being available to answer questions about their products.

Finding one-on-one time to talk with a doctor may be easy for patients (though some of you may disagree) but not so for pharmaceutical representatives. How could they educate the doctor on the miracles of their wonder drug if they couldn't even talk to him? After all, most doctors are busy seeing patients or completing administrative tasks usually into and through their lunch hours (or more often the case, lunch minutes). To get the doctor's attention, some pharmaceutical companies began to entice doctors for their time, and more than free samples were being left behind.

In the days of yesteryear, physicians would be offered compensation for their sit-down time with these representatives.

Compensation was often indirect with simple "gifts" ranging from pens to sticky notes labeled with the pharmaceutical company or medication name. Drug lunches became commonplace as the offer of free food was used to draw physicians out of their offices to eat a bite or two during their lunch hour. Outright bribes and kickbacks in the way of vacation travel and offers of company stock have even been reported. As you can imagine, these tactics could heavily influence what medications a healthcare provider would choose to prescribe.

It could be argued that by giving free samples the pharmaceutical companies are offering a service. They are not making but actually losing money by giving the product away. Some may go so far as to say they are not affecting a doctor's prescribing habits because the doctor is not pulling out their Rx pad to write an actual prescription. The doctor is only handing out samples.

The reality is something quite different.

What does the doctor do when free samples of a specific medication are no longer available? He could change to another medication but if a patient is satisfied with the initial product, he could well write out a prescription for that medication. When considering prescription options for other patients, that brand name would be one of the first that comes to mind given his close proximity and experience with the medication. This doesn't necessarily mean that will be the final prescription written out for the pharmacy, but it does come into consideration. Time and again doctors will say that they are not influenced by interactions with the pharmaceutical industry but some studies have shown otherwise.

Think about what this could mean for your health. If your provider is directly or indirectly influenced to prescribe certain medications and starts you on a more expensive medication, this will affect your out-of-pocket costs. It could affect your everything.

I am proud to have gone through a family medicine residency program at the University of Connecticut where the residents in training were not allowed to speak directly with pharmaceutical representatives. All interactions with the pharmaceutical representatives were supervised by a staff pharmacist to assure that only objective data was shared between all parties and that no gifts of any kind were exchanged. This sort of training allowed me to keep perspective not only through my medical training but beyond into my clinical practice.

The ACA now takes those reigns. The Physician Payments Sunshine Act provision of the ACA requires that payments to healthcare providers greater than $10 per gift or greater than $100 per year be reported to the government. The results will be available to the public online at a future date and you may be interested to see if your doctor makes the list or not.

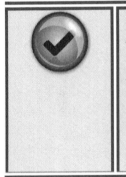

FACT CHECK:

The Affordable Care Act limits the amount of gifts a pharmaceutical company can offer to healthcare providers and will develop a web site to allow you to see if your healthcare provider accepted gifts over the allowed amount.

Failure to adhere to the mandatory reporting will result in fines to the pharmaceutical company. Fines may be as high as $1,000 to $10,000 per infraction but could reach as high as $10,000 to $1,000,000 over a year if it is proven that data was intentionally withheld.

The Physician Payments Sunshine Act does not mean that free samples go away. Free samples, medication vouchers and rebate cards are not considered gifts according to this new law. What it may mean is reduced face time for the representatives with the doctors, which may well be a good thing as the information provided is likely biased in some way. It is salesmanship after all.

Decreasing the influence of the pharmaceutical companies on prescribing habits could also encourage healthcare providers to favor generic medications over brand-name ones. The end result could be reduced costs for the healthcare system at large.

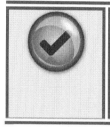

FACT CHECK:

The Affordable Care Act does not consider free samples, medication vouchers or rebate cards to be gifts.

Most medication samples are for brand-name medications, not generic ones. These samples tend to be the newest to the market and for that reason tend to be the most costly. Most of these medications are placed on tier 2 and above on insurance formularies and have the highest copays.

Given their limited supply, healthcare providers tend to reserve free samples for the most needy, those who cannot afford their medications. Still, sometimes the distribution of these samples may include other groups of people looking for a deal. The cost savings for the patient who receives free samples is obvious.

Free samples are a clever marketing device. Once the samples are no longer available, patients will often be prescribed these higher-cost medications with higher out-of-pocket costs. A doctor may offer a different set of medications, either an alternative free sample or a less expensive prescription medication, but that is a disruption to the patient's care. New medications risk new side effects. Will the new medication be as effective as the old one? Changes to a medication regimen require trial and error and close monitoring, which could lead to increased frequency of doctor visits and other healthcare costs.

As you see, there is good and bad that comes with using free samples. The ugly takes the shape of a donut hole.

The Donut Hole

Before you start to drool over the possibility of a delicious bakery treat, remember that I am a doctor first and foremost so put down the donut (and pick up a piece of fruit)! What we are looking at here is not a sweet ball of fried dough but the gaping hole it leaves behind, the missing piece. The "donut hole" is the gap in the coverage of prescription medications through Medicare.

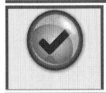

FACT CHECK:

Donut or Doughnut?

I am from New England.

It is a very interesting concept and one that leaves many seniors baffled as they try to manage their healthcare costs. I will do my best to explain it to you.

1. **Medicare Part D Coverage (Up to $2,850)**
2. **Donut Hole ($2,850-$4,550)**
3. **Catastrophic Coverage ($4,550 and over)**

Depending on your Medicare Part D plan, you will first pay out a deductible. Once this dollar amount has been spent, Medicare Part D will begin to cover the cost of your medications. For each prescription you fill, you will pay a copay. The cost of the copay depends on the tier of medication as discussed earlier. The higher the tier, the higher the copay. Your Part D plan covers the difference in the cost of the medication left behind after your copay. This coverage continues until you and your Part D plan have spent $2,850 (at least this is the value set for 2014). This limit will change annually.

FINE PRINT:

Costs Counting Toward the First $2,850 (Pre-Donut Hole)

- Annual deductible
- Copays and coinsurance
- What Part D pays for your medications

It is important to understand what is included up to that point. The $2,850 includes the cost of your deductible, your copays and the dollar amount spent by Medicare to cover the remaining costs of your medications. What it does not include are cost expenditures for your monthly premiums or for any medications not covered on your Part D formulary. Also, medications purchased outside of the United States do not meet criteria. I am talking to you Canadian mail-order!

When you and Medicare reach that $2,850 limit, the cost of your prescription medications increases significantly.

Welcome to the donut hole.

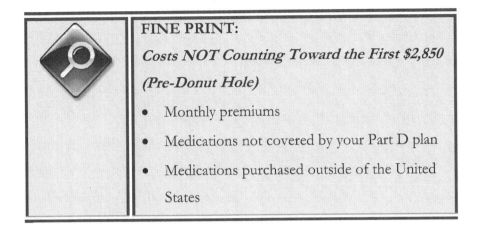

FINE PRINT:

Costs NOT Counting Toward the First $2,850 (Pre-Donut Hole)

- Monthly premiums
- Medications not covered by your Part D plan
- Medications purchased outside of the United States

It is a dark place where I have seen far too many people struggle not only with their finances but their health. People who have had their medical conditions stabilized on their medication regimens may no longer be able to afford them. They may have to cut other expenses in their life, hopefully not in the way of food, housing expenses or necessary utilities. They may opt to stop their medications altogether (please, don't do this!). More commonly, their healthcare providers may offer them other less expensive medication options until the coverage gap closes. As discussed previously, there is no guarantee that the medication changes will work out. More monitoring may be required during the transition and this could add other costs.

Medicare Part D and its coverage gap came into existence in 2003. Since enactment of the ACA in 2010, there have been improvements that have decreased the cost burden to Medicare beneficiaries although costs remain high. Instead of paying a smaller fixed copay, you will pay an outright percentage of costs for your medications. You will not pay the retail price of the medications because prices have been negotiated between your Part D plan and the pharmacies, whether it is a traditional store or a mail-order pharmacy. This decreases costs to a certain extent but the blow to your wallet may be bigger than you anticipate.

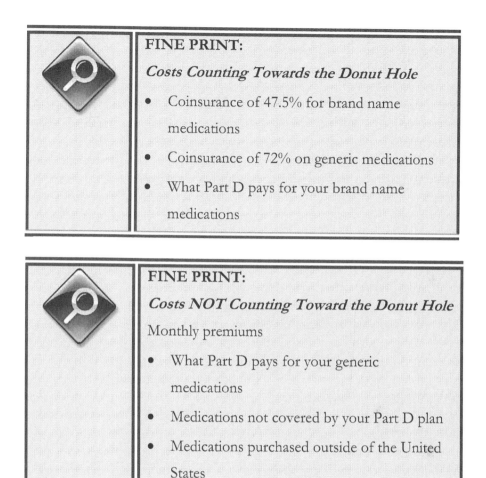

FINE PRINT:

Costs Counting Towards the Donut Hole

- Coinsurance of 47.5% for brand name medications
- Coinsurance of 72% on generic medications
- What Part D pays for your brand name medications

FINE PRINT:

Costs NOT Counting Toward the Donut Hole

Monthly premiums

- What Part D pays for your generic medications
- Medications not covered by your Part D plan
- Medications purchased outside of the United States

You will spend 47.5% of the negotiated price on brand name medications and 72% on generic medications. This means that 52.5% and 28%, respectively, of your medication expenses are covered by Medicare. The percentage you pay on generic medications will decrease to 25% by 2020.

Take a moment to consider when I told you about the monthly cost of ENBREL and HUMIRA. Retail costs were a whopping $2,700 to $2,900 per month. In this scenario, what could have been an $80 dollar copay for a high-tier medication may now cost the patient more than $1,200 for a one month supply. Of course, the actual dollar amount of the copay or coinsurance will vary depending on the Medicare Part D plan someone has selected as well as what price the pharmaceutical company negotiated with the insurance.

The donut hole continues until one of two things happen: 1) the end of the annual Medicare calendar year is reached or 2) your prescription costs reach $4,550. That means you could be caught in the donut hole for as much as a hearty $1,700 (donut-hole end $4,550 minus donut-hole start $2,850) before you can get additional coverage.

Your coinsurances count towards the $1,700. The dollar amount that Medicare spends on your brand-name medications counts towards the $1,700 but the amount they spend on your generic medications will not. Again, your monthly premiums and non-formulary medications are not counted towards the $1,700.

FINE PRINT:

The donut hole begins at $2,850 and ends at $4,550.

Once the donut hole closes, you enter the phase of catastrophic coverage. Doesn't that sound delightful? At least the name acknowledges that by this point you have been saddled with an obscene amount of expenditures.

During catastrophic coverage, your spending reduces to smaller copays or coinsurances depending on the specific Part D plan you selected. For 2014, catastrophic coverage will cost either $2.55 for generic medications (or $6.35 for brand-name drugs) or 5% of the total cost of the medication, whichever cost is greater.

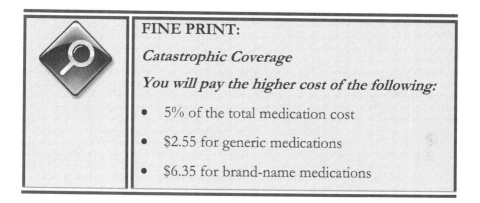

FINE PRINT:

Catastrophic Coverage

You will pay the higher cost of the following:

- 5% of the total medication cost
- $2.55 for generic medications
- $6.35 for brand-name medications

Why Have a Donut Hole?

If the donut hole has proven to be such a heavy financial burden for American seniors and other Medicare beneficiaries, why does it exist at all? The answer is simple: cost containment.

Ultimately, it would be ideal if each Medicare beneficiary did not have to pay for prescription medications at all. Even better, not to need the medications at all. Back to that good old philosophy of diet, exercise and positive thinking. Relying on that alone unfortunately is not realistic with the aging body and conditions that sneak in by virtue of our genetic makeup.

What the donut hole does is incentivize healthcare providers to keep costs in mind as they prescribe to their patients. Favoring cheaper medications to more expensive ones, their choices may decide whether a person reaches that coverage gap in the first place. Also, when and if the gap is reached, the costs to that person will be less because the medications in and of themselves are more cost-conscious: tens of dollars out-of-pocket for a generic medication versus hundreds to thousands on a brand-name.

What would happen if there were no financial constraints put on prescription costs? Would there be excessive amounts of brand-name medications prescribed at higher cost? Would pharmaceutical companies gain the upper hand with their advertising and marketing campaigns? Would people demand brand-name medications because of it? I know this may sound irrational. Why would someone demand a brand-name before trying a reasonable generic alternative? You would be surprised how that prestige factor I mentioned earlier sneaks its way in. I have treated quite a few people with that mindset, who all but demand to try a certain medication because they believe it to be the best of the best. Those marketing campaigns work.

I will let you in on a not-so-secret secret. Generic medications are likely your best bet. They are the tried and true. These medications are available as generics because they have been around for many years. They have stood the test of time. The newer medications may have been approved by the FDA with clinical data to support their use but they do not have the years of experience to back them up. If you think about it, I am sure you could name quite a few medications that have been removed from the market for safety reasons in recent years. The prestige may rightly belong to the generic, and not the brand-name, products.

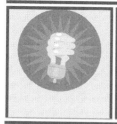

CONCEPT:

Generic medications have more years of clinical data and may be safer than some newer brand-name medications.

Healthcare costs are on the rise and the government is trying to prepare its resources. With the Medicare population increasing in size every year, they are trying to explore ways to decrease spending from the Medicare Trust Fund. It is not solely to save money but to preserve Medicare for future generations. You can almost see why they are going about it this way just as easily as you can see they are going about it all wrong.

The problem with the donut hole, among other things, is that those with the most complicated diseases or a compilation of medical conditions literally pay the most, almost as if they are penalized for being ill. They may have more needs, require more prescriptions. Perhaps they have failed to respond to generic medications and more expensive medications must be used to stabilize their health. There really ought to be a better way to do this. Health should be preserved for all.

Medicare Part B Medications

Prescription drug coverage is not limited to Part D. Part B does offer some allowances though its coverage is very limited. Coinsurances are frequently required.

Certain vaccinations are covered under Medicare Part B. For those who qualify, these include influenza (flu), pneumococcal (pneumonia) and hepatitis B vaccines. Flu shots are covered once every flu season for everyone. Pneumonia shots are offered one time only. Hepatitis B shots are offered only to those considered at high risk. High risk factors to consider are diabetes, end stage renal disease, hemophilia, past transfusion of blood products and healthcare workers at risk for exposure. Shingles vaccination is covered under Medicare Part D, not Part B.

FINE PRINT:

Hepatitis B vaccinations may be covered only if you are considered high risk.

Also covered under Part B are medications that require the use of durable medical equipment. Examples are medications used in nebulizer machines and medications used in infusion pumps.

Medications that require administration by a licensed medical provider are generally covered under Part B as well. Injectable medications administered by you or other persons may include the following if certain conditions are met:

- Blood clotting factors for hemophilia
- Erythropoisis-stimulating for anemia caused by end stage renal disease and other specific conditions
- Intravenous immunoglobulin for primary immune deficiency disease
- Intravenous nutrition and tube feeding
- Medications for post-menopausal osteoporosis

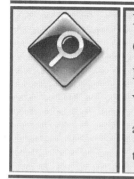

FINE PRINT:

Certain medications will only be covered under Part B for very specific conditions.

Your healthcare provider must document the appropriate diagnosis or Medicare will not cover the costs.

Note that some of these medications require very specific diagnoses—here's where medical necessity comes into play. If a man needs an injectable osteoporosis medication, he is out of luck simply because he doesn't have a pair of X chromosomes. Medicare Part B will not cover the costs because osteoporosis alone is insufficient as a diagnosis and he obviously has not experienced menopause. Post-menopausal osteoporosis must be clearly specified for Part B coverage. He will have to rely on his Part D coverage or otherwise pay out of pocket even if his bones are equally as weak as a woman suffering in her menopausal years. Likewise, if the doctor prescribing the medication does not clearly delineate her condition as post-menopausal when he prescribes it, the woman may equally be charged for the medication.

Part B coverage of medications taken by mouth is even more restricted.

- Anti-nausea medication used within 48 hours of a chemotherapy regimen at strengths available in intravenous form
- Anti-cancer medication at strengths available in intravenous form or as a prodrug or activated version of the intravenous medication

People with renal failure or end stage kidney disease may also be eligible for Part B coverage of specific medications. For those who have had a kidney transplant, Medicare will provide Part B coverage for the immunosuppressant medications needed to prevent the body from rejecting the organ.

After 36 months, some of these transplant patients will lose their Medicare coverage if they no longer meet the criteria for renal failure. After all, they now have a functioning kidney and do not meet disability status. This is an unfortunate situation because they will still need to pay for these immunosuppressant medications for the rest of their lives.

For coverage to continue, the patient needs to qualify for Medicare by the traditional eligibility standards of age or disability. Coverage of these medications requires that the transplant has taken place in a Medicare-certified facility.

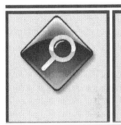

FINE PRINT:

After 36 months, you may lose your Medicare coverage if your transplanted kidney is working and you are less than 65 years old.

Part B coverage may even be used when you stay overnight in a hospital. This may seem confusing if you recall that Part A covers hospital expenses (another example of the fine print). Part A covers for inpatient care and Part B for outpatient care. Aren't you inpatient if you are IN the hospital? Not necessarily. We will save that discussion for Chapter 8.

In addition to prescription medications, Medicare covers a percentage of the cost for other items used in the home, if it considers these items medically necessary (there's that magic phrase again). Medical necessity is a key concept to understand and one that can set off more than a little debate. There is no all-inclusive list made available to the public, or to healthcare providers for that matter, that states what Medicare defines as medically necessary in every situation. If you come across such a list, please be sure to let me know—I want a copy.

FINE PRINT:

Medical supplies and equipment may only be covered if Medicare considers them medically necessary.

Your healthcare provider needs to prescribe these items according to a specific medical diagnosis. Without a defined medical condition, most certainly the item will not be considered necessary in Medicare's judgment. The more specific the diagnosis, the more likely it will meet Medicare criteria. For example, leg pain may not warrant use of crutches but a fracture of the left tibia may do it.

Medicare will often send forms to your doctor's office that request certain questions be answered before they decide whether to cover your expenses. There is little room here for describing your personal circumstances. The questions are generally in yes/no or numerical format, i.e., a test result. If coverage is later denied based on the answers, a doctor may write an appeal letter on your behalf to see if they can convince Medicare that the prescription was medically necessary.

Part B covers the majority of outpatient utilities and requires a coinsurance be paid, usually at 20% cost.

Ambulance services may be covered if deemed medically necessary because other means of transportation would be considered unsafe or threatening to your health. For example, driving yourself to a hospital in the middle of a heart attack would pose a risk not only to you but to the public at large. However, you cannot choose what hospital you go to. You will be brought to the nearest available facility even if the hospital you usually use is one minute further away in distance. You will pay the full cost of the ride if you request the other facility. Paramedic care may also be billed to the ambulance service.

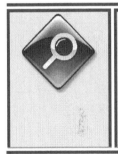

FINE PRINT:

Ambulance services are covered, if medically necessary, to the nearest available facility (hospital or skilled nursing facility) which may or may not be the facility of your choice.

There are people who abuse the use of the ambulance. Ambulances are not medically necessary to bring you to appointments, even if those appointments are for your health. Medicare will not cover the cost and you will receive a large bill. It will save you money to do some research and find local resources that may provide you free transportation. You can call your healthcare provider, the local American Red Cross or even your Town Hall to find information about services where you live. In the worst case scenario, it would even be better to call for a taxi cab than to foot an ambulance bill.

According to the Centers for Disease Control, 10.9 million Americans over the age of 65 had diabetes in 2010. Part B covers many of the diabetic supplies needed to manage the condition. These may include insulin syringes and insulin needles. Glucometers to measure your sugar, control solutions to make sure the meter is working, lancets to prick your finger and tests strips to collect the blood sample are all included. Do not take this to mean that you can check your blood sugar as much as you want. Based on the specific diagnosis your doctor provides (you would be stunned to know how many there are for diabetes), Medicare may set restrictions on how many supplies per month are covered. How well controlled your sugars are and whether or not you use insulin also comes into the equation.

If you are on insulin, you may be allowed 100 test strips and lancets per month. If you are not on insulin, that will extend to the same number of supplies over three months unless your doctor specifically documents a medical need.

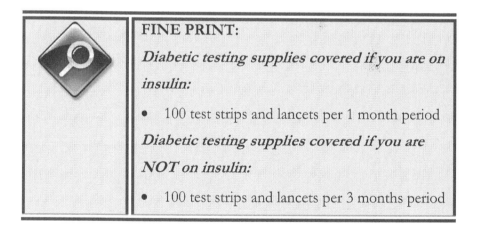

FINE PRINT:

Diabetic testing supplies covered if you are on insulin:

- 100 test strips and lancets per 1 month period

Diabetic testing supplies covered if you are NOT on insulin:

- 100 test strips and lancets per 3 months period

Durable medical equipment is defined as equipment for the home that is intended for long-term use. There are a variety of supplies that may be covered under Part B.

Respiratory supplies may range from home oxygen to continuous positive airway pressure (CPAP) machines for sleep apnea. Nebulizer machines may also be covered.

Orthopedic supplies may include braces, shoe inserts, crutches, walkers and canes, though interestingly not white canes for the blind. A white cane designates a type of cane used by the visually impaired to help sense the environment around them. The white signifies to the public that the person using the cane is blind. Other covered items may include wheelchairs, both standard and motorized, and prosthetic devices.

For those with special needs, hospital beds, air mattresses, hydraulic lifts and bedside commodes may be indicated. Other supplies include infusion pumps, suction pumps, feeding pumps and ostomy supplies.

Please know that this is not an exhaustive list.

Ms. Jones Treats Her Medical Condition

Ms. Jones has diabetes and she uses two different medications to keep her sugars from getting too high. Part B will pay for her diabetic supplies, up to 100 test strips and lancets every three months, while Part D will offer coverage for her medications. Generics will require a lower copay than brand name medications.

The only problem is that her sugars have been rising higher more recently even though she has been doing everything right. She has been taking her medications as prescribed and has been eating a proper diet. Her doctor has begun to discuss the possibility of starting insulin. As much as she dislikes the idea, her doctor has discussed the potential complications of diabetes if her sugars continue at these higher levels. She agrees to start insulin.

While on insulin, she will be required to check her sugar levels more frequently. This is essential to ensure her sugar levels do not drop too low. She is now eligible to receive more diabetic supplies than she had previously, up to 100 test strips and lancets per month. Her doctor now has to change the prescription to reflect this diagnosis change or the added costs may be shifted to the patient.

Hopefully, Ms. Jones will not spend more than $2,850 (premiums excluded) over the course of the year for medications covered by her Part D plan. If she does, she will be pushed into the donut hole, a not so tasty treat, until she spends a total amount of $4,550. At that time, she will become eligible for catastrophic medication coverage.

Chapter 5 – Medicare and Provider Visits

Ms. Jones wants to make sure she is in good health. After all, stopping diseases in their early stages or preventing them altogether can sometimes mean the difference between life and death. When she heard that health check-ups and screening tests were now free under Medicare, she made an appointment with her doctor.

It always amazes me how people read only what they want to read. The fine print just disappears into the background when the word "free" crosses the page or screen. Take a buy one, get one offer for example: maybe you buy more than you need because you think you are getting a bargain. Really you are just being coerced into buying something in the first place. Free is rarely free. You have to read on to see what you are really buying into.

What's In a Visit?

"Let your heart feel for the afflictions and distress of everyone, and let your hand give in proportion to your purse."
— *George Washington*

Yes, it is true. You are offered a Welcome to Medicare Visit and it is FREE. You are offered an Annual Wellness Visit every year after that and it too is FREE. The Affordable Care Act has applauded itself time and again over adding this preventive medicine opportunity for its Medicare beneficiaries as well it should. These are wonderful offerings if you know how to use them to your benefit.

BUT...

Before you get overly giddy rubbing your hands together at the free sticker, let me first ask you a simple question. What does a visit mean to you? This may seem like a rhetorical question but I need you to really think about it.

Wiktionary.com defines visit, the noun, as:

1) A single act of visiting
2) (medicine, insurance) A meeting with a doctor at their surgery or the doctor's at one's home.

Is this more or less what you were expecting? One could think of a visit in a casual sense, a meeting where two people get together. This could be for a simple chat or talk. In medical terms, however, there are more implications. Meeting with a doctor implies an inspection or examination of some kind, although it would be nice to think that your doctor's bedside manner could also qualify as a chat or talk. The truth is these free visits offered to you by Medicare lean more to the talking variety than you may think.

Your expectation and the reality of what will happen at your visit may be skewed. Both of these visits, the Welcome to Medicare Visit and the Annual Wellness Visits, do not include the doctor laying hands on you. There is no examination included.

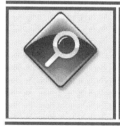

FINE PRINT:

The Welcome to Medicare visit and Annual Wellness visits do NOT include a physical examination.

Some people may find this surprising. After all, how can a medical visit intended to prevent disease not include a listen to your heart and lungs? How can a physician find cancer if he does not examine a woman's breast or a man's prostate? While all these components may be important to early identification of disease, they are not the true intention behind these Medicare visits. Instead, these visits stand as a foundation from which to pursue the recommended screening interventions. Essentially, it is intended to be a consultation visit for discussion only.

This is where the nomenclature gets sticky. The word "visit" too often becomes interchanged with exam. Quite frankly, the office staff can sometimes be as confused as the patients scheduling appointments. In this case, though, the words do matter. It is not surprising when given the medical context. So when you sign up for your Welcome to Medicare "exam", know that you may be waiting for a long time—since it does not exist.

The Welcome to Medicare Visit

This visit is offered to you once and only once within the first year after signing up for Part B. This is the case whether or not you signed up at eligibility age. Covered under Part B, the visit itself is free but some of its individual components—in particular, screening tests that may be ordered at the visit—may not be.

First and foremost, your healthcare provider will sit down with you to discuss your history. To do a thorough job, this takes dedicated face time. Let us look to see what should be included.

- **Medical History** – This should include a review of your medical problems, past and present, including surgeries. You are the only you. Understanding your personal health history to this point in your life will help guide your provider towards the most appropriate treatment and screening options.

- **Medication History** – Understanding the purpose for each medication and how it interacts with your other medications is very important to minimize side effects. This includes not only prescription medications but over-the-counter medications as well. You would be surprised how many over-the-counter products, even certain vitamins, can interfere with your prescription drugs. To make the most of your visit, it is helpful for you to bring your medications in with you to your appointment.

- **Family History** – You may be at higher risk for certain conditions based on your genes. Your healthcare provider should review your family history and specifically ask about medical conditions that tend to be inherited. This discussion will determine if you are at risk for certain diseases and again will guide treatment and screening options.

- **Social History** – We are not talking about going to cocktail parties here, though that could be part of it. Your social history essentially addresses your lifestyle choices. Use of tobacco products, alcohol and drugs will be discussed. Your degree of physical activity will be taken into consideration. This is not an exhaustive list but stands as an opportunity for your healthcare provider to counsel you on lifestyle choices that could improve your health.

Vital signs are also an important part of any visit. Your healthcare provider or her nursing staff may be the one to take these measurements though this may be the only laying on of hands you get during the visit. This includes measuring your height, weight and blood pressure. Your height and weight are used to calculate a number known as the body mass index (BMI) that categories your weight into underweight, normal weight, overweight or obese. Again, this is used as a tool to determine your health risk.

A simple vision screening test should also be performed at this visit. Do not confuse this to mean a full glaucoma screen. This screen may be as simple as reading an eye chart. Poor vision is a risk factor for falls and this is intended as a general safety assessment.

Your healthcare provider should also discuss your mental health and screen for depression. Depression is all too common and quality of life can be improved if the condition is identified early and addressed, either by counseling or medication if necessary.

It is not always easy to talk about advanced directives, i.e., end of life plans. The Welcome to Medicare Visit encourages you and your provider to discuss this in an open forum. It is not required that you make any final decisions at the visit but understanding your options is key to planning for your future.

Based on all this information gathering, your provider will now discuss with you what screening tests may be appropriate for you as an individual. You will be given a written list of tests that Medicare offers to you. Some of these screening tests may have costs attached. A detailed review of these preventive services will be discussed later in the chapter.

The Annual Wellness Visit

Annual Wellness Visits are offered through Part B after you have been on Medicare for 12 months. This is not based on a calendar year but on an actual 12 month calendar. That is to say, having an Annual Wellness Visit one year in September and then the next in August is not covered. The visits must have at least 11 months between them. It is not required that you have had the Welcome to Medicare Visit in order to take advantage of these annual preventive visits.

This visit is essentially an extension of the Welcome to Medicare Visit as there is significant overlap between the two. Any changes to your personal history are reviewed. Vital signs are rechecked. Your preventive screening options are again outlined.

There are two features that make these visits distinct from the Welcome to Medicare Visit. The first of these is the health risk assessment or HRA. This is a questionnaire for you to complete that reviews topics ranging from your dietary habits to depression screening to safety in your home. Your healthcare provider may mail this questionnaire to you in advance for completion or you may complete it once you attend your visit. The HRA is an important tool to determine your health risks. It is also a mandatory component of the visit in order for Medicare to cover the provided services.

The second component of the Annual Wellness Visit involves screening for cognitive impairment. According to the Alzheimer's Association, 5.2 million people had Alzheimer's disease in 2013 and the disease remains the sixth leading cause for death in our country. Memory loss, confusion and dementia may be a result of Alzheimer's disease but many other conditions could be the cause. The truth is that the risk for cognitive impairment increases as we age and this affects how we respond to our environment. It becomes a matter of safety. The Annual Wellness Visit offers your healthcare provider the opportunity to screen you for any changes to your cognitive status on a yearly basis. Medicare does not specify how your provider ought to complete the screening, only that screening is indicated. There are many approaches a provider may take to complete the screening. That said, do not be too surprised if you are asked a lot of odd questions or are asked to draw a clock.

The one aspect of your Welcome to Medicare Visit that is not continued in your Annual Wellness Visits is a vision test. This is unfortunate since vision tends to get worse as you get older. One would think vision tests should be covered annually for safety reasons but to no avail. Your healthcare provider may offer you a vision test at your Annual Wellness Visit but be aware that it may not be free of charge.

Other Covered Provider Services

"Ankles are nearly always neat and good-looking, but knees are nearly always not."

— Dwight D. Eisenhower

Part B covers the cost of doctor visits both inpatient and outpatient—more on this in Chapter 7. It also covers services offered by other providers. This section will review the most common situations where you will use outpatient provider services.

Physical Therapy (PT), Speech-Language Pathology services (SLP) and Occupational Therapy (OT) are services frequently required for those who suffer from orthopedic problems, rheumatologic problems, strokes and other disabling conditions. Part B covers for these outpatient services with a 20% coinsurance (you pay 20% of the visit cost) if it deems these therapies to be medically necessary. There are those magic words again. Your therapist plays a key part in determining what is medically necessary.

The amount that Medicare will pay is limited. Therapy limit caps have been set for 2014 at $1,920 for Physical Therapy and Speech-Language Pathology services combined and for $1,920 for Occupational Therapy on its own. Starting in 2014, services received in a critical access hospital (CAH) were also included in the therapy limit cap. The therapy limit cap includes the amount you pay as a coinsurance as well as the amount Medicare pays, i.e., the remaining 80%. If you had not used your Part B deductible for other healthcare needs, it would be included in this amount as well. In a way, the therapy cap resembles how the donut hole works except there is no end to the hole here, just a drop off. After the therapy cap has been reached, you will be responsible for all subsequent costs.

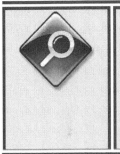

FINE PRINT:

Therapy Cap Limits

- Physical Therapy (PT) and Speech-Language Pathology (SLP) services (combined) = $1,920

- Occupational Therapy (OT) = $1,920

To get a sense of these costs, Healthcare Bluebook estimates the charge for an initial Physical Therapy visit to be $147 and follow-up visits at $80. Of course, this will vary based on what services are actually provided at those sessions. Some therapists use different techniques and equipment such as ultrasound, massage and traction that may add extra fees for any given visit. Because of this variability, I would look to these Healthcare Bluebook estimates more as a minimum baseline cost in this scenario. It can be a very reliable guide, however, for other healthcare costs such as laboratory tests, imaging studies and surgical procedures.

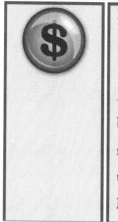

HELPFUL HINT:

Healthcare Bluebook

www.healthcarebluebook.com

A free website and smartphone/tablet app, owned by CAREOperative, LLC, that provides local and national cost estimates for common healthcare tests and procedures.

Make sure you are getting a fair deal.

Defining medically necessity lies in the hands of the therapist providing your services. They must carefully state the reasons their services are appropriate and necessary for your recovery and clearly document this in your medical chart for each visit. It is possible that the therapy cap could be waived if Medicare approves of their reasoning. However, know that your chart will be flagged for an automatic Medicare audit if your services exceed $3,700 for combined Physical Therapy and Speech-Language Pathology services or for Occupational Therapy services.

Mental health services are often necessary to treat a range of psychiatric conditions. Counseling and therapy services are covered at a coinsurance of 20% if they are provided by a qualified healthcare professional in an outpatient setting (not during an inpatient hospitalization). Qualified professionals include physicians, physician assistants, nurse practitioners, certified nurse-midwives, clinical nurse specialists, clinical psychologists or clinical social workers.

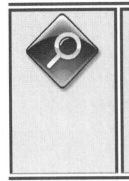

FINE PRINT:

Medicare Audit

You will automatically be flagged for a Medicare audit if your combined PT/SLP or OT costs exceed $3,700, even if your therapist has deemed the services medically necessary.

Advance Beneficiary Notice of Non-Coverage

It is important that you discuss the costs for any tests or procedures performed with your healthcare provider. This is especially true for Physical Therapy, Speech-Language Pathology Services and Occupational Therapy since there is a risk that Medicare may not consider them medically necessary. In fact, your provider has an obligation to tell you if there is a risk that Medicare will not cover the costs of tests or procedures that are being ordered.

This information should be provided to you in written form as an Advance Beneficiary Notice (ABN) of Non-Coverage and given to you BEFORE any test or procedure is completed. You will be required to sign this form as acknowledgement that Medicare may not pay for certain services. In effect it becomes a contract stating that you agree to pay any charges not covered by Medicare. If you choose not to sign the ABN, the healthcare provider reserves the right not to proceed with services. For obvious reasons, he wants to get paid. If he forgets to have you sign one, he is out of luck.

If an **ABN** is not given to you in advance of the tests and procedures provided and Medicare does not pay for the services, you are **NOT** financially liable for the cost of the studies. I repeat, you are **NOT** financially liable.

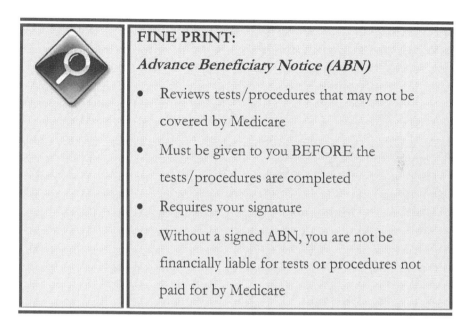

FINE PRINT:

Advance Beneficiary Notice (ABN)

- Reviews tests/procedures that may not be covered by Medicare

- Must be given to you BEFORE the tests/procedures are completed

- Requires your signature

- Without a signed ABN, you are not be financially liable for tests or procedures not paid for by Medicare

I will add a caveat here. Some healthcare providers may have you sign an informed consent form for a procedure instead of an official ABN. It may make mention of possible non-coverage of the test within that form. If you sign it, you may be responsible for the costs, even if there is not a formal ABN. Always read any document before you sign and ask questions if there is anything on it you don't understand.

Keep in mind, however, that there is a distinction to be made between the healthcare provider ordering a test and the one actually performing the test. What this means is that your provider may order a test but if he does not it is not perform it in his office, he is not the one required to offer you an ABN. The provider or facility that completes the test is the one responsible. Simply stated, your healthcare provider is responsible for what he does, not for what others do.

The most common example of this occurs with blood work. Your healthcare provider may send you to a laboratory facility to have tests drawn. The laboratory facility is obligated to provide you with an ABN because they are the one taking the risk that they will not be paid for their services. Likewise, when a provider refers you to a specialist for care, the specialist becomes responsible for any tests or procedures he performs.

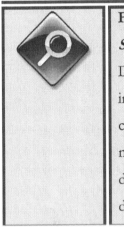

FINE PRINT:

Screening vs. Diagnostic Colonoscopy

Did your provider have you sign an ABN (or an informed consent form that discussed what is covered) before your screening colonoscopy? If not, you may not be liable for the costs of a diagnostic colonoscopy if one became necessary during the procedure.

In the case of a colonoscopy, the provider performing the study must offer you the ABN. This becomes especially important when it comes to screening colonoscopies. As you will learn in the following chapter, a screening colonoscopy may be converted to a diagnostic one if an abnormality is found during the procedure. The difference is that the screening colonoscopy is outright free to you and the diagnostic colonoscopy requires you to pay a Medicare coinsurance. If the person performing the study does not provide you with an ABN to discuss the possibility for a diagnostic colonoscopy BEFORE the procedure is completed, you will not be liable for those extra costs.

Medicare Penalties

"There's only so many priorities that you can fund. What you choose to target, you need to win."

— *John Hancock*

Everyone likes a bargain but at what cost?

It frequently happens that a person will ask their healthcare provider to perform additional services at their Welcome to Medicare Visit or their Annual Wellness Visit. After all, it saves him time from having to come to the office for another visit. The healthcare provider may agree to do this, if time allows, but this person must be aware that he may be charged the cost of an extra visit.

If you attended one visit, how can you be billed for two? As you recall, the Welcome to Medicare and Annual Wellness Visits are free. Medicare specifically outlines what services are to be provided at these visits. Any additional services are not covered and require another visit be billed to accommodate them. In this scenario, even if you have scheduled one of the free Medicare visits, you could also be billed a copay for a traditional office visit.

I can already hear the grumbles because I have literally heard them in the past. The provider is obviously "trying to make a buck". I can assure you that is not the intent. The intent is to avoid Medicare fraud and fines. Let me explain.

Medicare reserves the right to randomly audit charts in a medical office. The purpose for this is to reduce fraud. As sad as it is, there have been excessive abuses to the system in the past and

Medicare has recovered billions of dollars by ramping up audits and investigations.

When billing errors are noted in a chart, Medicare fines the provider for the infringement but on a larger scale, a percentage scale. For example, if Medicare audited 10 charts and found 1 chart with errors, they assume that 1 out of every 10 charts had a billing error. Medicare will then fine the provider based on 10% of his total Medicare patients. If the average patient panel is 2,000 patients, that can lead to excessive fines. One error can lead to a heavy financial burden for a medical office.

The Medicare Fraud Strike Force was established in 2007 and for good reason. Far too many people are abusing the system to take hard earned dollars away from Medicare funds. One shocking case in 2007 exposed 481 fake companies in Miami that were billing Medicare for durable medical equipment with charges of $237 million in 2006. In 2011 alone, the federal government recovered $4.1 billion in fraudulent charges.

While allowing you to have a follow-up visit at the same time as a Wellness visit may not seem to be a dastardly deed, Medicare still does not want to give away something for nothing. You pay nothing for the Welcome and Wellness visits but Medicare is paying your provider on the back end. That is to say, your provider bills Medicare for services rendered. After an audit, Medicare may not acknowledge the visit you received as one of the covered Welcome or Wellness visits and may penalize that healthcare provider or its office for billing as such. Medicare may do this by denying your provider payment for the visit, subjecting the office to fines or otherwise. How Medicare chooses to address these issues is, and may always be, a work-in-progress but trust me, your provider does not want to get on Medicare's bad side. It puts his entire medical practice at risk.

It can be all too easy to demand more from your healthcare provider but you must understand that they have as much to gain or lose as you do when it comes to Medicare's evolving processes. It is more important that you establish a healthy physician-patient relationship and discuss with them any concerns you have. Your provider should equally be open about what he can and cannot do. Together, hopefully you can learn what works best for both of you.

Ms. Jones Wants a Physical Exam

Ms. Jones attended her Welcome to Medicare Visit. Her healthcare provider, Doctor B. Good, took the time to carefully review her medical history and learned that not only did she have diabetes but that she also had a history for high cholesterol. She had smoked a half pack of cigarettes per day for 5 years but quit more than a decade ago. She is not sexually active and has not been for more years than she can count. She has never had a blood transfusion. Her family history is notable for diabetes but no other medical conditions.

Her vital signs were checked, showing that her blood pressure was high and her weight put her into the obese category with a BMI of 31. She passed her vision test with flying colors. There was no sign of depression after screening. Together, she and Dr. B. Good also discussed advanced directives, her plans for end of life care.

When she asked about a physical exam, Dr. Good explained that this was not included as part of the Welcome to Medicare Visit.

She was surprised but decided she would have an exam performed at her next follow-up visit.

With all this information gathered, Dr. Good reviewed that Medicare would offer specific preventive services to her based on her history. Let's take a good hard look at what that will include in Chapter 6.

Chapter 6 – Medicare and Outpatient Services

Ms. Jones attended her Welcome to Medicare Visit and her Annual Wellness Visits one year apart. At each visit, Dr. B. Good reviewed her medical history and risk factors. Armed with this information, he reviewed the tests he recommended to screen for disease.

How the doctor wants to screen and what Medicare will cover may not be in alignment. Understanding what tests are covered, what they are looking for and how they will help your healthcare provider to offer you better care is key to getting the most out of Medicare. This chapter outlines the outpatient services Medicare covers and at what cost.

FINE PRINT ALERT!!!

FINE PRINT ALERT!!!

FINE PRINT ALERT!!!

Preventive Screening for Cardiovascular Disease

Cardiovascular disease is more than prevalent in our society. It includes diseases such as coronary artery disease, congestive heart failure, angina, hypertension, aortic aneurysm and stroke among other conditions. According to the Center for Disease Control, there were 597,689 deaths from heart disease alone in 2010. This was the leading cause of death in the United States that year. Doing what we can to minimize these diseases plays a major role in keeping you healthy and may reduce healthcare costs for the future, for both you and the healthcare system at large.

Medicare appreciates the importance of screening for risk factors that could lead to cardiovascular disease. For one, blood pressure screening is performed at every Annual Wellness Visit free of charge. Based on these results, your healthcare provider may counsel you with diet and lifestyle recommendations to reduce your blood pressure. This becomes an opportunity to discuss whether medication options are appropriate for your situation.

FINE PRINT:

Blood pressure screening and counseling are free of charge as part of your Welcome to Medicare and Annual Wellness Visits.

The amount of fat in our bodies can contribute to blockage of arteries, possibly leading to heart attack and stroke. Part B coverage allows for screening of cholesterol, lipids and triglycerides once every five years. For accuracy, this test is best performed when you are fasting if possible.

Medicare does not take into consideration whether or not you already have known cholesterol or lipid problems. Part B covers the screening test free of charge only once every five years. Any additional lipid screenings required in between those time periods will be charged to Part B as a non-preventive service. Depending on what diagnosis your healthcare provider links to those additional tests, Medicare may or may not cover the cost of the test. Examples of covered diagnoses include coronary artherosclerosis, diabetes, essential hypertension, heart failure, hypertriglyceridemia, mixed hyperlipidemia, pure hypercholesterolemia, obesity and transient cerebral ischemia.

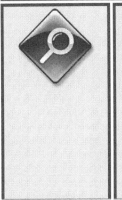

FINE PRINT:

Cholesterol, lipid and triglyceride screening

- Free of charge once every 5 years
- Any additional screenings performed in < 5 year intervals may be covered by Medicare only if linked to a proper diagnosis by your healthcare provider

FINE PRINT:

Costs of blood and laboratory tests

1) Cost of collecting the blood specimen

ASK YOUR PROVIDER IF THE COST CAN BE WAIVED IF IT IS PERFORMED IN THEIR OFFICE

2) Cost of processing the blood specimen in the laboratory

It is important to understand the added costs of blood tests. First, there is the cost of collecting the blood from your veins. This requires needles and test tubes and skilled personnel to gather the sample. Second, there is the actual cost of processing the blood sample in the laboratory. Part B may offer coverage for the latter and not the former, though Medicare may cover this cost if it is for a test considered medically necessary.

If the blood draw is done in your healthcare provider's office, it may be possible for the office to waive the draw fee. Every office will have a different protocol and you won't know if you can find cost savings here unless you ask. Your provider does not have the authority to ask an outside laboratory facility to waive this fee.

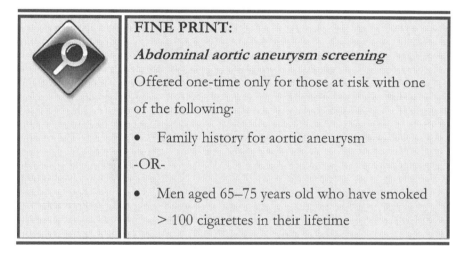

FINE PRINT:

Abdominal aortic aneurysm screening

Offered one-time only for those at risk with one of the following:

- Family history for aortic aneurysm

-OR-

- Men aged 65–75 years old who have smoked > 100 cigarettes in their lifetime

Abdominal aortic aneurysm screening is performed by ultrasound. The ultrasound looks to see if your aorta is larger than it should be. Once it reaches a certain size, it may be at risk for rupturing, which could be fatal. Part B offers a screening ultrasound one-time and only to people it considers at risk. The risk factors Medicare outlines are very specific. The first of these considerations is if there is a known family history for aortic aneurysms. The second is gender specific. For men between the ages of 65 and 75 years old, those who have smoked 100 or more cigarettes in their lifetime are considered at risk.

Preventive Screening and Services for Diabetes

According to the Center for Disease Control, 20.9 million Americans had diabetes in 2011. Of these people, 41.8% were 65 years of age and older. Complications of diabetes are varied but all too common. The high sugars associated with diabetes can attach to small- and large-sized blood vessels. This can lead to lead to heart and kidney disease. Your vision may be impaired when sugars collect on the retina. Nerve damage or neuropathy can develop causing pain or numbness.

Part B allows for screening of diabetes if certain conditions are met. High blood pressure, high cholesterol, high triglycerides, high sugar levels and obesity, defined as a BMI > 30, may be associated with a diagnosis of diabetes.

Other risk factors for diabetes include age greater than 65 years old, being overweight (BMI 25–30), or having gestational diabetes. Diabetes in pregnancy is frequently associated with diabetes later in life. Mothers with infants born at weights greater than 9 lbs may have had glucose problems during their pregnancy, even if they passed their gestational diabetes screening. A family history for diabetes may contribute to risk for developing diabetes as well. Any two of these factors will qualify for diabetes screening.

Medicare does not specify how to screen for diabetes. Diabetes screening may be done with a simple fasting glucose blood test: levels greater than 126 are used to diagnose diabetes. Non-fasting glucose levels may be suggestive for the disorder if they are greater than 200. Some healthcare providers may use a blood test called the hemoglobin A1C. Levels greater than 6.5 are indicative of diabetes. An oral glucose tolerance test measures your body's response to sugar by measuring your blood sugar before and after ingesting a fixed amount of glucose; this test is somewhat labor intensive.

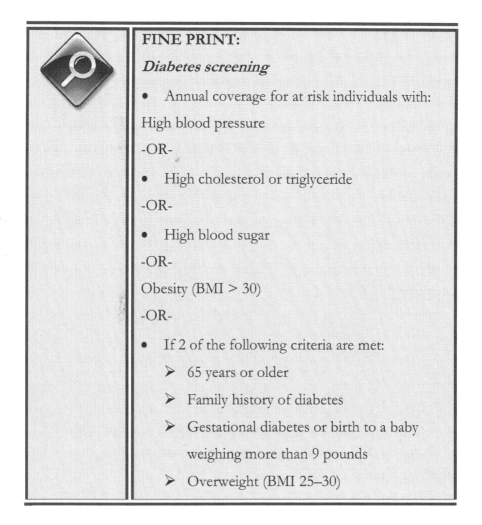

FINE PRINT:

Diabetes screening

- Annual coverage for at risk individuals with:

High blood pressure

-OR-

- High cholesterol or triglyceride

-OR-

- High blood sugar

-OR-

Obesity (BMI > 30)

-OR-

- If 2 of the following criteria are met:
  ➤ 65 years or older
  ➤ Family history of diabetes
  ➤ Gestational diabetes or birth to a baby weighing more than 9 pounds
  ➤ Overweight (BMI 25–30)

For those confirmed to have diabetes, it is important to understand how to best manage the disease to minimize complications. Part B covers diabetic self-management training to educate diabetic patients about the disease. This training may include information about a diabetic diet, how to check blood sugar levels and for those requiring insulin, how to appropriately inject insulin. Part B covers up to 10 hours of initial training if sessions are ordered by a healthcare provider. In subsequent years, Part B will cover up to two extra hours per year in group sessions of 2–20 people for sessions lasting 30 minutes or more. If group sessions are not locally available or if a provider indicates a medical reason why group sessions would not be appropriate, for example psychiatric reasons, an exception can be made to the requirement. Each visit requires a coinsurance payment of 20%.

FINE PRINT:

Diabetes Self-Management Training

20% coinsurance for each visit

- Initial training: Up to 10 hours in one year
- Follow-up training: Up to 2 hours per year
    - Group sessions of 2–20 people
    - Sessions for a minimum 30 minute duration
    - Must be in a new calendar year than initial diabetes training

Preventive Screening and Services for Infection

Infectious diseases are essential part of preventive medicine. The spreading of disease becomes a public health issue. Medicare has targeted specific infections for coverage.

The United States Preventive Screening Task Force announced its recommendation in June 2013 to screen for hepatitis C in people at high risk for the disease or for people born between 1945 and 1965. In March 2014, Medicare agreed to include this screening in its preventive services. People at high risk include those who have ever used injected illicit drugs or who received a blood transfusion before 1992. Annual screening is covered for those who continue to use illicit drugs. For those not considered at high risk but who were born between 1945 and 1965, screening is offered one time only. An epidemiologic study found a higher prevalence of hepatitis C in this age group.

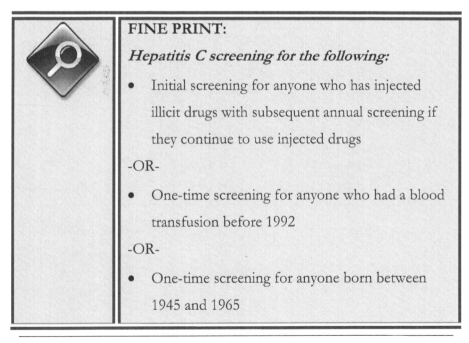

FINE PRINT:

Hepatitis C screening for the following:

- Initial screening for anyone who has injected illicit drugs with subsequent annual screening if they continue to use injected drugs

-OR-

- One-time screening for anyone who had a blood transfusion before 1992

-OR-

- One-time screening for anyone born between 1945 and 1965

Sexually transmitted infections (STI) include chlamydia, gonorrhea and syphilis. Hepatitis B may be an STI although it can also be transmitted in other ways. Other STIs are not specified by Medicare and may not be covered. These may include herpes and mycoplasma infections among other infections. Part B covers screening of the specified STIs once annually for sexually active Medicare beneficiaries who are considered at risk. Risk factors are not clearly defined by Medicare but may include unprotected sexual intercourse with multiple partners and partner infidelity.

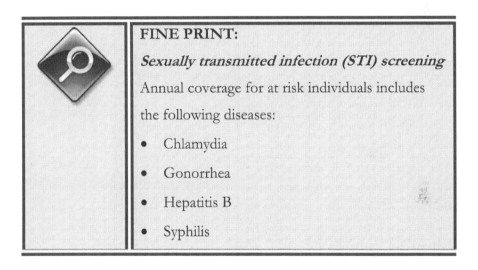

FINE PRINT:

Sexually transmitted infection (STI) screening

Annual coverage for at risk individuals includes the following diseases:

- Chlamydia

- Gonorrhea

- Hepatitis B

- Syphilis

Taken one step further, those at risk may continue to be at risk if steps are not taken to change their behaviors. Medicare Part B covers behavioral counseling sessions to address these issues. Up to two separate face-to-face visits may be covered for up to 30 minutes per session. This counseling is covered in the outpatient setting but is not covered as a preventive service if the counseling is performed in the hospital or in a skilled nursing facility. In those settings, charges will apply.

Human immunodeficiency virus or HIV may be more common than you think. In 2009, the Centers for Disease Control reported that 1.1 million Americans were infected with HIV and as many as 200,000 of them unaware they even had the virus. Medicare Part B covers HIV screening once annually for any Medicare beneficiary at risk and for any who simply request the test.

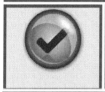

FACT CHECK:

In 2009, 1.1 million Americans had HIV with more than 200,000 of them unaware of the fact.

Pregnancy is considered a special scenario. After all, the mother's health is not only at risk but also that of the baby. Medicare Part B covers STI and HIV screening over the course of the pregnancy.

Though much controversy has sprung up over vaccinations in recent years, vaccinations have been proven to save lives and decrease the spread of infection. Medicare covers flu shots, pneumonia shots and hepatitis B shots for appropriate candidates. The details of this are discussed in Chapter 4 under "Medicare Part B Medications".

Preventive Screening for Colorectal Cancer

The CDC reports that more than 131,600 people were diagnosed with colorectal cancer in 2010 and more than 52,000 died from the disease. In the United States, colorectal cancer is the third most common cancer across both genders and remains the second leading cause of cancer death. Medicare appreciates this major health concern and offers different screening strategies to look for the disease.

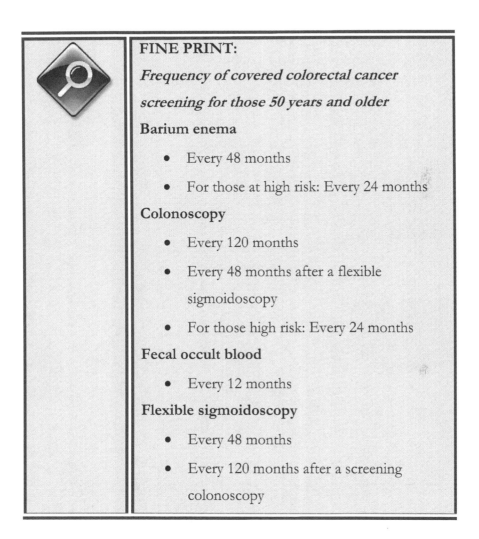

FINE PRINT:

Frequency of covered colorectal cancer screening for those 50 years and older

Barium enema

- Every 48 months
- For those at high risk: Every 24 months

Colonoscopy

- Every 120 months
- Every 48 months after a flexible sigmoidoscopy
- For those high risk: Every 24 months

Fecal occult blood

- Every 12 months

Flexible sigmoidoscopy

- Every 48 months
- Every 120 months after a screening colonoscopy

Screening opportunities begin at age 50 for both men and women. Each test has different risks associated with it. Your healthcare provider will guide you towards the best option for screening depending on your medical history.

A simple rectal examination performed in the office can be used to check for blood in the stool. Alternatively, your provider may supply you with "stool cards" to collect samples of your stool at home and bring back to the office for analysis. This screening is known as a fecal occult blood test. A positive result could be indicative of underlying colorectal cancer though many other conditions could cause blood in the stool as well. This is the least invasive testing and can be checked once annually free of charge. If it is positive, your healthcare provider will likely recommend additional screening with another test. Please note that a negative screening test does not exclude a diagnosis of colorectal cancer.

Flexible sigmoidoscopy and colonoscopy are more invasive but provide the most information. A camera is inserted into the rectum and used to directly visualize the colon. Sigmoidoscopy extends only to the lower part of the colon whereas colonoscopy extends further into the colon. When used for screening purposes, these tests are free under Medicare Part B.

However, do not be surprised if you end up with a bill just the same. In the case that a suspicious area is detected during the examination and intervention is pursued, such as a biopsy, the study is no longer considered a screening test—it becomes a diagnostic one. You will now be responsible to pay a cost for the procedure at a 20% coinsurance.

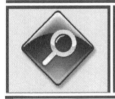

FINE PRINT:
Your screening colonoscopy could be converted to a diagnostic colonoscopy during the procedure.

There is no way to know in advance if you will require a diagnostic procedure. After all, isn't that why screening is being performed in the first place? To not pursue the intervention would be foolhardy, as you would need to go through another vigorous round of testing to confirm what could have been completed in the first go round. One and done, I say.

However, if you have had colon polyps in the past, there is a high probability that they will be detected again. Colon polyps are common and they can be precursors to cancer. You are at higher risk for a screening colonoscopy being converted to a diagnostic one if you have a proven history for polyps. Then again, it is possible that a diagnostic colonoscopy could be planned from the get-go if you have the diagnosis on your record. This is something you should discuss with your provider before the study.

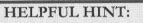

HELPFUL HINT:

Ask your healthcare provider in advance if you are scheduled for a screening or diagnostic colonoscopy.

The frequency of screening will vary based on which test is pursued. For those at normal risk, flexible sigmoidoscopies and colonoscopies may be performed every 48 months or 120 months, respectively. If a colonoscopy was performed previously, it could be followed up by a flexible sigmoidoscopy in 120 months. If a flexible sigmoidoscopy was performed previously, it could be followed up by a colonoscopy in 48 months. For those at higher risk for colorectal cancer, colonoscopies may be pursued every 24 months.

If your risk for complications is considered too high for either procedure based on your medical history, your provider may recommend an alternative test called a barium enema. A barium enema inserts dye into the rectum via an enema and looks for irregular shapes or narrowing on x-ray that could be suggestive for colon cancer. Like the fecal occult test, positive results may be suggestive for colorectal cancer but not diagnostic.

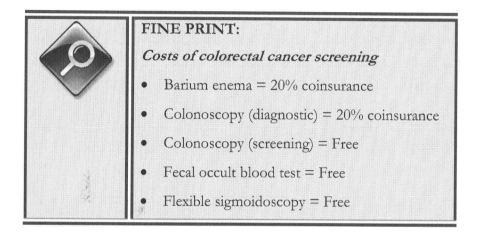

FINE PRINT:

Costs of colorectal cancer screening

- Barium enema = 20% coinsurance
- Colonoscopy (diagnostic) = 20% coinsurance
- Colonoscopy (screening) = Free
- Fecal occult blood test = Free
- Flexible sigmoidoscopy = Free

Preventive Screening for Women

With the advent of Pap smear screening, cervical cancer rates have considerably declined over the years. The CDC reports that more than 11,800 women were diagnosed with cervical cancer in 2010 while more than 3,900 women died from the disease in the same year.

Part B covers cervical and vaginal cancer screening with a Pap smear and a manual pelvic exam. Pelvic examinations enable the healthcare provider to assess the vulva, the vagina, the uterus and the ovaries. These services are covered every 24 months (2 years) for all women and every 12 months (1 year) for women if they meet high risk criteria. These high risk criteria may include a woman being of childbearing age or having an abnormal Pap smear test result within the last 36 months (3 years). Pap smear screening is not indicated for women who have had their cervix removed by way of a hysterectomy.

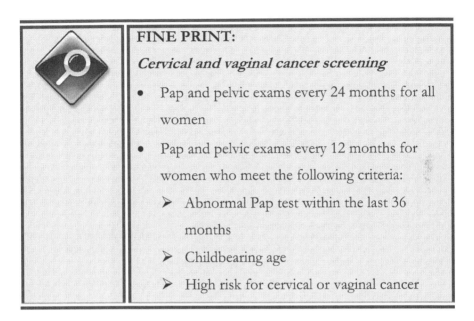

FINE PRINT:

Cervical and vaginal cancer screening

- Pap and pelvic exams every 24 months for all women
- Pap and pelvic exams every 12 months for women who meet the following criteria:
  - ➤ Abnormal Pap test within the last 36 months
  - ➤ Childbearing age
  - ➤ High risk for cervical or vaginal cancer

Breast cancer is the most common non-skin cancer in women according to the CDC. In 2010, approximately 207,000 women and 2,000 men were diagnosed with breast cancer while approximately 41,000 women and 440 men died from the disease. Clinical breast exams are covered every 24 months (2 years) under Medicare Part B. Mammograms, however, have become the standard for identification of early breast cancer.

A woman becomes eligible for a baseline mammogram screening between the ages of 35 and 39 years old. At 40 years old, she becomes eligible for routine screening every year. Medicare covers the cost of screening mammograms but a coinsurance of 20% is required for diagnostic mammograms. The imaging modalities are different in that diagnostic mammograms may have better resolution to look at a suspicious area of tissue. A diagnostic mammogram may be indicated if looking at a suspicious breast mass or for following someone who has had a history for breast cancer. Medicare does not cover ultrasounds or MRIs as preventive screening options for breast cancer.

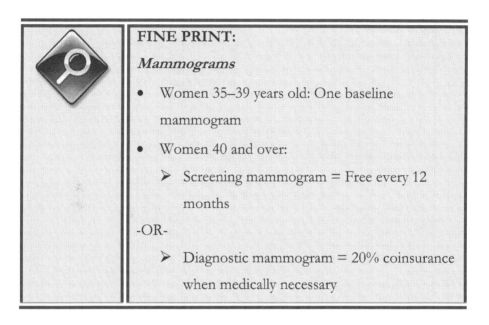

FINE PRINT:

Mammograms

- Women 35–39 years old: One baseline mammogram

- Women 40 and over:

    ➢ Screening mammogram = Free every 12 months

-OR-

    ➢ Diagnostic mammogram = 20% coinsurance when medically necessary

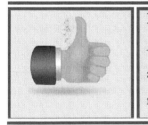

HELPFUL HINT:

Ask your healthcare provider in advance if you are scheduled for a screening or diagnostic mammogram.

Similar to screening and diagnostic colonoscopies, how your provider orders the test will determine how much you pay. You have the right to know. Be proactive and ask how the study is being ordered.

Preventive Screening for Men

Prostate cancer is the most common non-skin cancer in men according to the CDC. In 2010, more than 196,000 men were diagnosed with prostate cancer while more than 28,500 men died from the disease.

Screening for prostate cancer has become more controversial in recent years. Debates have been waged on whether early detection of prostate cancer actually saves lives. In particular, the prostate specific antigen (PSA) test has been questioned as a viable screening tool because studies have shown it may lead to too many false positive results. These false positive results may lead to unnecessary testing and complications. The PSA is a simple blood test that measures a protein that is secreted by the prostate. Other screening tests are in development but have not yet been approved for coverage by Medicare.

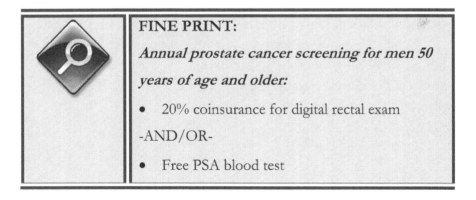

FINE PRINT:

Annual prostate cancer screening for men 50 years of age and older:

- 20% coinsurance for digital rectal exam

-AND/OR-

- Free PSA blood test

Part B covers prostate cancer screening every 12 months. This may include a PSA screen covered free of charge or a digital rectal exam which requires a 20% coinsurance. The digital rectal exam allows your healthcare provider to actually feel the prostate to see if it is enlarged or has any suspicious masses on it suggestive for cancer.

Other Covered Preventive Screening and Services

Osteoporosis is a disease that weakens bones and increases your risk for fracture and disability. Part B covers screening of osteoporosis by way of bone density studies. These studies are covered every 24 months (2 years) if certain risk criteria are met.

For women, menopause is the most common cause. Estrogen generally protects the bones and when it decreases during menopause, the bones lose their strength. Other medical conditions that decrease estrogen will have a similar effect. Long-term use of steroid medications such as prednisone can also lead to thinning of the bones. Hyperparathyroidism is a hormonal condition that may leech calcium out of bones, triggering osteoporosis. When x-rays suggest weakened bones or fractures of the vertebral spine, a bone density study may be indicated to confirm the diagnosis. Bone density studies may be required to monitor how well the bones are responding to treatments for osteoporosis.

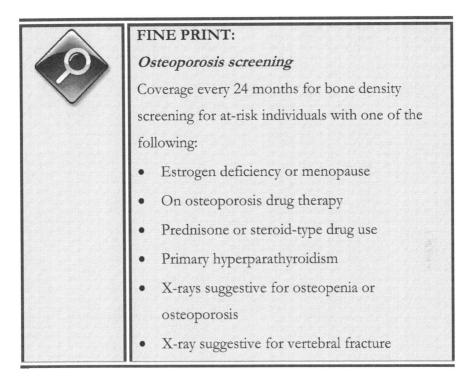

FINE PRINT:

Osteoporosis screening

Coverage every 24 months for bone density screening for at-risk individuals with one of the following:

- Estrogen deficiency or menopause
- On osteoporosis drug therapy
- Prednisone or steroid-type drug use
- Primary hyperparathyroidism
- X-rays suggestive for osteopenia or osteoporosis
- X-ray suggestive for vertebral fracture

Part B covers screening and counseling for certain conditions. Tobacco use has serious health consequences ranging from heart disease to lung disease to cancer. The list goes on and on. Benefits of smoking cessation can be seen immediately as well as in the long-term. Medicare recognizes the impact that smoking has on your health and offers coverage for eight one-on-one sessions of smoking cessation counseling over a 12 month period. These visits may review the consequences of smoking, an overview of behavioral interventions and considerations for medications to help you quit smoking, if appropriate. These visits come at a cost of a 20% coinsurance.

Alcohol overuse, similar to tobacco, can lead to an array of health complications, heart disease and liver disease to name a few. Steps taken to identify an abuse problem can help to mitigate these healthcare issues. Part B covers alcohol abuse counseling as a free preventive service annually.

Depression not only impairs quality of life but has been associated with heart disease. Part B covers annual depression screening free of charge once per year.

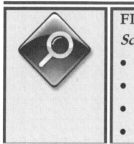

FINE PRINT:
Screening and counseling
- Alcohol abuse screening and counseling
- Depression screening
- Obesity counseling for those with a BMI > 30
- Tobacco use cessation counseling

Obesity counseling is offered to those with a BMI greater than 30 without needing to pay. This may include discussions about diet, exercise and medical conditions that could be contributing to obesity. Behavioral modifications may be encouraged and the possibility of interventional medications reviewed.

Medicare also covers one-on-one nutrition counseling or medical nutrition therapy with a registered dietician or other certified professional for those with diabetes, kidney disease or both. Kidney disease includes those on dialysis and those who have received a kidney transplant within the past 36 months. In order for Part B to cover this as a preventive service, a referral must be placed by your healthcare provider. If you make the appointment on your own, expect to pay for the visit.

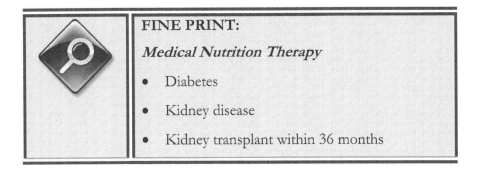

FINE PRINT:

Medical Nutrition Therapy

- Diabetes
- Kidney disease
- Kidney transplant within 36 months

What Your Provider Wishes Were Covered

I wish I could say that there were more preventive services offered through Medicare. The unfortunate truth is that the offerings, as good as they are, are limited. It may well be that your healthcare provider recommends additional tests and studies that Medicare may not cover based on your underlying conditions.

For example, the United States Preventive Screening Task Force (USPSTF) announced its recommendation in December 2013 to screen for lung cancer in people between the ages of 55 and 80 years old who are considered at higher risk for the disease. Specifically, the USPSTF has advised for low-dose CT scans in these individuals. In May 2014, Medicare declined to include these CT scans under its preventive care umbrella.

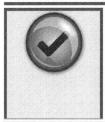

FACT CHECK:

Medicare will not cover lung cancer screening by low-dose CT scan even though it is recommended by the USPSTF for high-risk individuals.

Throughout this book you have seen kidney disease mentioned time and again. Obviously, Medicare appreciates this to be a major health issue with serious consequences. The CDC estimates that 10% of Americans have some degree of chronic kidney disease and that risk for disease increases with age. While certain factors may increase your risk for kidney disease, such as high blood pressure or diabetes, as much as 28% of kidney disease arises from other causes. Despite this fact, Medicare does not include blood tests to check your kidney function under its preventive services umbrella.

This does not mean that Medicare won't cover the tests at all. They may be covered if your healthcare provider attaches the order to a medical condition that you have. Some examples of approved diagnoses are diabetes and chronic kidney disease. As we have discussed in previous chapters, your healthcare provider must take care to select a Medicare approved diagnosis code for that particular test or the costs will not be covered.

HELPFUL HINT:

Medicare Coverage for Other Laboratory Tests

(Not on the Preventive Screening List)

Medicare may cover the costs of other tests if your healthcare provider attaches the order to an approved diagnosis.

Kidney function is easily checked with simple and inexpensive blood tests. One of these is the serum creatinine test. According to the Healthcare Bluebook, the national average out-of-pocket cost for a serum creatinine test is $23. The test may be ordered on its own but is commonly included among a panel of tests, commonly referred to as chemistries or metabolic panels. Oddly enough, these panels are often less expensive than ordering the tests separately. If your healthcare provider does not offer one of these tests to you, I would encourage you to ask for it. It is very important to know that your kidneys are in working order.

There are many other tests that your healthcare provider may want to order for you. Some common tests are listed below.

- Anemia becomes all too common as we age for a variety of reasons, whether it be from malnutrition or a vitamin deficiency or even a warning sign that you are bleeding internally. Hemoglobin levels may be screened for directly with a $39 price tag or as part of a complete blood count for $23. Some offices even have a finger prick test that may cost you even less.

- The liver is an essential organ that controls your metabolism. Knowing whether your liver is working appropriately is important, especially for those who take medications that must be processed by the liver. Liver function tests average $24.

- A thyroid-stimulating hormone (TSH) test at $23 is used to screen for hypothyroidism, a condition that increases with age and that could result in abnormal heart rhythms and weight gain.

All of these costs are out-of-pocket expenses only if Medicare does not accept any of the cost responsibility. Again, if your provider attaches a diagnosis that Medicare approves for the test, you may have little or no cost. A 20% coinsurance would average $4.50 for each of the tests listed above.

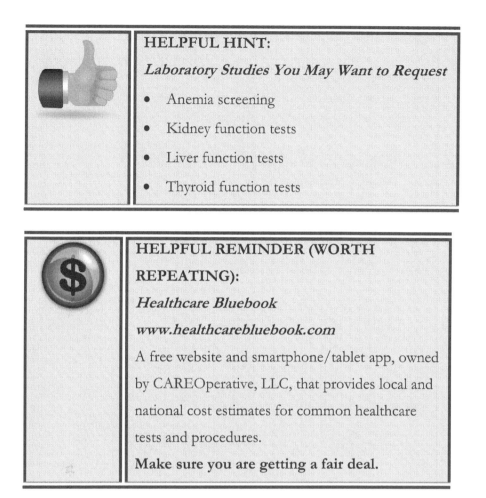

HELPFUL HINT:

Laboratory Studies You May Want to Request

- Anemia screening
- Kidney function tests
- Liver function tests
- Thyroid function tests

HELPFUL REMINDER (WORTH REPEATING):

Healthcare Bluebook

www.healthcarebluebook.com

A free website and smartphone/tablet app, owned by CAREOperative, LLC, that provides local and national cost estimates for common healthcare tests and procedures.

Make sure you are getting a fair deal.

Ms. Jones Gets Her Preventive Checklist

Ms. Jones attended her Welcome to Medicare Visit. After a thorough discussion, Dr. B. Good reviewed with her what preventive studies Medicare would cover. He also reviewed why she may not have been eligible for other studies. The final preventive checklist provided a care plan that was tailored to her needs. Remember she has diabetes.

Cancer Screening

Service	Eligible	Reasoning
Fecal Occult Blood Test	Yes	She opted to take stool cards home to complete annual testing.
Colonoscopy	Yes	She chooses colonoscopy over other available tests for colon cancer screening.
Mammogram	Yes	She is due for her first annual mammogram.
Pap & Pelvic Examination	Yes	She is due for her first Pap & pelvic examination and then every 24 months.

Cardiovascular Screening

Service	Eligible	Reasoning
Aortic Aneurysm Screening	No	She does not have a family history for aneurysm.
Lipid Screening	Yes	She is due for her first lipid screening now and then every 5 years.

Diabetes Services

Service	Eligible	Reasoning
Diabetes Self-Management Training	Yes	She meets criteria for initial training up to 10 hours in a year.
Medical Nutrition Therapy	Yes	Her history for diabetes meets criteria.

Infectious Disease Screening and Services

Service	Eligible	Reasoning
Hepatitis C Screening	Yes	She is allowed one-time screening based on her age.
HIV Screening	Yes	She is low risk but requested screening.
STI Screening	No	She is not at high risk.
Vaccination – Influenza	Yes	Annual shots are covered during flu season.
Vaccination – Hepatitis B	No	She does not have high risk factors.
Vaccination – Pneumonia	Yes	She is due for her one-time vaccination.

Other Available Services

Service	Eligible	Reasoning
Alcohol Abuse Screening and Counseling	Yes	If her annual screening is positive, her provider may proceed with counseling.
Bone Density Screening	Yes	As a postmenopausal female, she meets criteria for screening every 24 months.
Depression Screening	Yes	Included as part of the Wellness Visit
Obesity Counseling	Yes	She has a BMI > 30.

When she returned the next year for her Annual Wellness Visit, her weight was reduced, improving her BMI to 28. Her screening colonoscopy had returned with benign results. Her preventive screening eligibility for the subsequent year changed to the following:

Cancer Screening

Service	Eligible	Reasoning
Fecal Occult Blood Test	Yes	She opted to take stool cards home to complete annual testing.
Colonoscopy	No	She is not due for colonoscopy or flexible sigmoidoscopy for 9 years.
Mammogram	Yes	She is due for her annual mammogram if at least 11 months have lapsed between exams.
Pap & Pelvic Examination	No	She is not due for 12 months.

Cardiovascular Screening

Service	Eligible	Reasoning
Aortic Aneurysm Screening	No	She does not have a family history for aneurysm.
Lipid Screening	No	She is not due for another 4 years.

Diabetes Services

Service	Eligible	Reasoning
Diabetes Self-Management Training	Yes	She meets criteria for follow-up training up to 2 hours in a year.
Medical Nutrition Therapy	Yes	Her history for diabetes meets criteria.

Infectious Disease Screening and Services

Service	Eligible	Reasoning
Hepatitis C Screening	Yes	She already completed her one time screening.
HIV Screening	Yes	She is low risk and does not request screening.
STI Screening	No	She is not at high risk.
Vaccination – Influenza	Yes	Annual shots are covered during flu season.
Vaccination – Hepatitis B	No	She does not have high risk factors.
Vaccination – Pneumonia	Yes	She already received the vaccination.

Other Available Services

Service	Eligible	Reasoning
Alcohol Abuse Screening and Counseling	Yes	If her annual screening is positive, her provider may proceed with counseling.
Bone Density Screening	Yes	She is not due for 12 months.
Depression Screening	Yes	Everyone is offered annual screening.
Obesity Counseling	No	Her BMI is < 30.

Chapter 7 – Medicare in the Hospital

Ms. Jones slipped on a sheet of ice and landed on her hip. She had immediate pain and was unable to bear weight on her leg. She was rushed to the hospital by ambulance and found to have two fractures of her pubic bone. She had x-rays, CT scans, IV medications and consultation with an orthopedic surgeon. She stayed in the hospital overnight but the following morning, she was informed by the Case Manager that she was not considered an inpatient and would be responsible for a large percentage of the hospital stay costs.

What Defines an Inpatient?

"Everyone is stable at this time. If their condition appears to weaken, they will be brought to the hospital and either fed intravenously or nose fed."

— John Adams

What does it mean to be an inpatient? It may not be what you think because even the dictionary does not know the full meaning of the word, at least not according to the Centers for Medicare and Medicaid Services (CMS). To prove the point, let us look to wiktionary.org for the most commonly accepted definition:

inpatient *noun*

> A patient whose treatment needs at least one night's residence in a hospital; a hospitalized patient.

As a Medicare beneficiary, however, that definition is inadequate. Being IN the hospital, even for one night or more, is not enough to be considered an INpatient. To be an inpatient you need a whole lot more.

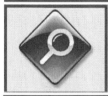

FINE PRINT:

You do not necessarily qualify as an Inpatient by virtue of staying overnight in the hospital.

There are two types of services you can be offered in the hospital. The first are outpatient services and the second are inpatient services. Staying in the hospital in and of itself is not sufficient to differentiate between the two. When you stay in a hospital overnight, you will either be placed under observation or admitted as an inpatient. It is important to know that observation services fall under the category of outpatient services.

FINE PRINT:

You will be either placed _Under Observation_ or admitted an _Inpatient_ for your hospital stay.

How can you be under observation when you are actively being evaluated in the hospital? The doctor is already providing you care. CMS interprets this observation period as a time when a person can be monitored to see if they will require inpatient services. Inpatient care is ordered only when the medical concerns are considered urgent enough to require direct hospital care.

A simple way to look at the difference between the two services is to see that outpatient services can be performed at any time. Outpatient studies can be performed anywhere—in a doctor's office, a department in a hospital or any healthcare facility. These studies may provide important information but can be performed non-emergently. Inpatient services require urgent evaluation for a condition that needs close supervision and monitoring. This may be a bit of an oversimplification but it relays the basic concept between outpatient and inpatient care.

Take the following example. A woman goes to see her doctor in the office about abdominal pain she had for several days. Her doctor suspects gallstones and orders an ultrasound. This is an outpatient study that can be performed in any Radiology department, whether that is in a hospital or not. He also orders some laboratory tests. She does not have to be admitted to the hospital to complete the evaluation. Her life is not at risk. If the doctor had concerns to this degree, he may have sent her to the hospital for a more urgent evaluation.

Another woman goes to the emergency room (ER) with the same symptoms. The ER doctor also suspects gallstones and orders laboratory studies and an ultrasound. If his concerns were for a severe or life-threatening condition, he may immediately admit her as an inpatient but often, until he has more information to guide his decision, he may place her under observation. That added information may include the results of the tests he ordered. If the tests return negative, she may be sent home to follow-up with her doctor in an outpatient setting for further evaluation. If concerning findings are found, she may then be admitted as an inpatient for continued care.

Again, this may be an oversimplification because in the brave new world of Medicare regulations, timing is everything.

The 2-Midnight Rule

On October 1, 2013, CMS implemented a change to Medicare that rocked hospital medicine to the core – the 2-Midnight Rule. You may have heard about it on the news. NBC Nightly News with Brian Williams has aired a series of exposés on the topic. The 2-Midnight Rule has drawn much negative media coverage, vilifying doctors and hospitals to a fault. The fingers may be pointing in the wrong direction. Doctors and hospitals are equally unhappy about the change. The American Hospital Association has gone so far as to sue the federal government questioning the lawfulness of the act.

The 2-Midnight Rule can be summed up as follows: Medicare will not consider a patient's hospital stay appropriate for inpatient coverage unless it is expected to span two midnights. This requires one of two conditions:

1) The doctor documents and justifies the expected timeline in the medical chart.

-OR-

2) The hospital stay actually crosses two midnights.

There are few exceptions to the rule.

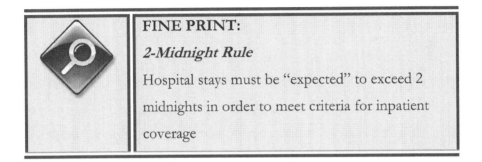

FINE PRINT:

2-Midnight Rule

Hospital stays must be "expected" to exceed 2 midnights in order to meet criteria for inpatient coverage

The two-midnight time stamp may seem arbitrary. By giving a formal definition, the government attempts to eliminate any shades of grey about timing. Unfortunately, this definition has also added a degree of unfairness to hospital admissions. Someone admitted at 11:59am will cross two midnights almost 24 hours sooner than someone admitted two minutes later at 12:01am. With most hospitals entering orders electronically these days, there is no way to bypass that time stamp. That first patient, even requiring identical care, may have a better opportunity to get inpatient coverage through Medicare.

Consider someone who has appendicitis. If a ruptured appendix is not removed, the patient could die. The medical services received in the hospital, appendectomy, are obviously medically necessary. Most people will go home the day after their appendix is removed if the surgical procedure does not have any unforeseen complications. This patient would be deemed appropriate for observation services under the new ruling whereas they would have been considered inpatient-appropriate prior to the 2-Midnight Rule.

Other factors come into consideration when deciding how a patient should be admitted. A doctor needs to document his level of concern for the patient, which could potentially override the 2-Midnight Rule, though there is no guarantee that Medicare will accept the doctor's rationale for the admission. The problem is that not all doctors document in the chart how long they expect a patient to stay in the hospital. Though they typically document a diagnosis and a care plan, doctors also need to write a statement that justifies why they think a patient is "expected" to stay more than two midnights. Without this documentation, the 2-Midnight Rule could remain unchallenged, with few exceptions.

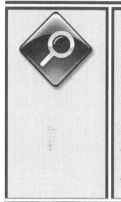

FINE PRINT:

Physician Documentation for Two Midnights

If a doctor documents a justifiable reason why a hospital stay is expected to exceed two midnights, he could potentially override the 2-Midnight Rule. There is no guarantee that Medicare will agree with the decision.

One would think that doctors could solve the two midnight conundrum by documenting a need for a two-midnight stay for all admissions. Even if the stay did not ultimately cross two midnights, Medicare may make an allowance based on the healthcare provider's documented concern. Unfortunately, doing this across the board would constitute fraud. The consequences of a Medicare audit could destroy a healthcare provider's career and bankrupt hospitals. What the 2-Midnight Rule does is strip power from the healthcare provider. Their medical judgment is, to a certain extent, set aside in favor of an arbitrary timeline.

To be clear, the 2-Midnight Rule does NOT mean that if you stay in the hospital longer than 2 days you automatically become an inpatient. Medicare will only cover for inpatient services if they consider them medically necessary. Yes, there is another hoop to jump through.

Medical Necessity

Evidenced-based medicine is all the rage as well it should be. Evidence-based medicine favors using information from medical studies rather than long-held beliefs that may not have data to back them up. Evidence-based medicine aims to improve the quality of medical care and to improve clinical outcomes for patients.

Medicare's bent towards medical necessity is essentially a call to evidence-based medicine. The tricky part is that Medicare does not tell us exactly what evidence-based medicine it likes to use and does not spell out other rules that meet its medical necessity requirements. The reality is that every clinical situation is different and it can be difficult to decide whether or not a case meets Medicare inpatient criteria.

This is the reason why companies have developed strategies to help guide hospitals in their admissions processes. McKesson is a large corporation that has built a line of products known as InterQual®[4] to

---

[4] InterQual is a registered trademark of McKesson Corporation.

help medical providers and hospital systems make clinical decisions about patient cases. The InterQual products are used by many managers and utilization reviewers across the country for use in their hospitals. You would be surprised by the subtle differences that can change a case from being appropriate for observation to being appropriate for inpatient status. Sometimes it is simply a matter of how fast IV fluid is being administered per hour.

FINE PRINT:

McKesson's InterQual products are used by many hospitals to determine appropriateness for inpatient admissions.

Sometimes, however, even the most well intentioned products will miss an inpatient case and call it appropriate for observation services. This is where a healthcare provider's medical judgment comes into play. Companies such as Executive Health Resources®[5] offer case reviews by board certified physicians across varied specialties. These physicians are trained in medical necessity compliance and assist hospitals in determining the appropriateness of inpatient admissions, according to available guidelines. Other companies may also provide similar services.

---

[5] Executive Health Resources is a registered trademark of Executive Health Resources, Inc.

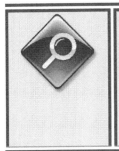
No method is perfect. Without full Medicare transparency on what they consider appropriate for inpatient criteria, even with InterQual products and physician peer-to-peer reviews, there will always be a risk that Medicare will decline a claim. This can lead to appeals and months or years waiting for a judicial review.

Observation and Inpatient Costs

One has to ask whether it really makes a difference if you are under observation or admitted as an inpatient. Your wallet definitely thinks so.

Someone who is admitted as an inpatient will have their hospital services covered by Medicare Part A. For every inpatient admission, there is a deductible of $1,216 that covers the first 60 days including hospital services, testing and medications. Medicare Part B services, however, will cover the physician fees. This requires the inpatient to pay a 20% coinsurance of the Medicare-approved cost for care provided by each medical provider. As discussed earlier, this applies only for healthcare providers who accept assignment. As reminder from Chapter 3, see the following fine print.

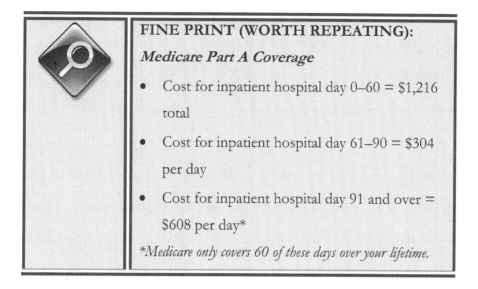

An individual placed under observation status will have his or her services covered by Medicare Part B, not Part A. Each service will be charged separately with a coinsurance or copay for each service. Physician services, as for inpatient status, will be billed at 20% of cost. The good news is that a single copay cannot cost more than the $1,216 that your Medicare Part A deductible would have cost you. The bad news is that your services added up together can far exceed this amount.

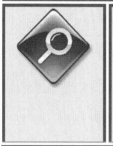

Depending on your length of stay and the specific services provided, it may be far less expensive to be an inpatient. When you are under observation, Medicare saves money by shifting more of the costs to you. It does not mean that Medicare does not want you to be an inpatient. Medicare wants you to receive inpatient care when they deem it appropriate. The hospital, however, may have a different set of objectives. They make more money when you are an inpatient because Medicare pays them a larger share of the cost. In this way, hospitals would actually prefer for you to be an inpatient whenever possible.

CONCEPT:

Hospitals tend to make less profit when you are placed under observation and would prefer you to be admitted as an inpatient.

To see how it plays out, let us use the example of appendicitis mentioned earlier in this chapter. A hospital may charge you differently based on whether you are under observation or admitted as an inpatient. According to Healthcare Bluebook, hospital services for an outpatient laparoscopic appendectomy average $8,141 nationwide (this cost does not include an overnight stay). An inpatient appendectomy, however, averages the same $8,141 for a 4-day stay (additional days would be charged at $1,800 per day and shorter stays at a cost reduction of $1,800 per day). You could potentially pay the same for a 1-day observation stay as a 4-day hospital stay. In other words, an observation stay costs $8,141 per day whereas an inpatient stay would cost only $2,741 per day. Keep in mind these numbers reflect what the hospital could charge you, not necessarily what would be paid by Medicare or another insurance. It's baffling that there would be any difference in cost for the same procedure.

Physician services and anesthesia services have similar charges regardless of your admission status, at least in this scenario. Healthcare Bluebook lists $1,152 as an average for physician fees and $730 for anesthesia services for the outpatient procedure and $1,227 and $724, respectively, for the inpatient procedure.

Because Healthcare Bluebook does not break down the specifics of the hospital services, it is difficult to estimate how much you would really pay if you were under observation in this example. These services may include the medical bed, medical supplies, IV therapy and laboratory fees among other items. At a minimum you would pay the $1,216 since a single copay cannot exceed the amount of the inpatient deductible but each hospital service will be billed separately. When the costs are broken down, you will pay far more than that. The sticker shock gets worse.

These costs are only national estimates and Healthcare Bluebook warns that there can be as much as 400% variation depending on where the services are provided. A study published in the Archives of Internal Medicine in 2009 reviewed cost differences between 19,368 appendectomies in California. For individuals between the ages of 18 and 59 years old who stayed in the hospital less than 4 days, costs ranged from $1,500 to $180,000! The average cost was $33,000. The costs varied widely even within the same cities, despite no surgical complications in these cases.

FINE PRINT:

Costs for the same services may vary widely across the country by as much as 400%.

California is not the only example. A September 2013 report from the Obama administration found similar cost variation nationwide. CMS reviewed the costs of hospital stays across 3,000 healthcare facilities for the 100 most commonly billed diagnoses. The differences were staggering. A joint replacement in Oklahoma cost

$5,300 whereas one in Monterey, California cost $223,000. Admissions for congestive heart failure ranged from $21,000 to $46,000 in Denver, Colorado and between $9,000 to $51,000 in Jackson, Mississippi. Of course, every patient situation is different but these cost differences are due to more than just particular health concerns. The system is rife with inequity.

An otherwise healthy 20 year old posted his hospital bill on social media after an appendectomy at Sutter Health in Sacramento, California in October 2013. His story went viral: the simple procedure cost him upwards of $55,000. The breakdown of his bill is seen in the table below. Even this is not a full detail of the charges. The individual lab tests, for example, are not broken down. Surely, more than one medical device was used. The doctor's fees are also not teased out from the other services provided.

	Full Charge	20% of Cost
Room and Board	$4878.00	$975.60
Pharmacy	$2420.56	$484.11 [$2420.56]
Laboratory	$1408.00	$281.60
Recovery Room	$7501.00	$1500.20 ($1216)
Medical/Surgical Supplies	$6428.75	$1285.75 ($1216)
CT Scan	$6983.00	$1396.60 ($1216)
Emergency Room	$2703.00	$540.60
IV Therapy	$1658.00	$331.60
Other Therapeutic Services	$210.00	$42.00
Anesthesia	$4562.00	$912.40
Operative Services	$16,277.00	$3255.40 ($1216)
TOTAL	$55,029.31	$10,368.36

No individual charge can exceed the amount of the inpatient deductible. This is the reason certain costs have the deductible amount listed in parentheses. Medicine (pharmacy) costs, are not covered by Part B. An individual under observation would be charged the full dollar amount of $2420.56 as listed in brackets.

Still, this case suffices as an example to show you how much an inpatient saves as opposed to someone under observation. Assuming a 20% copay and coinsurance for the services he received, an inpatient would pay a deductible of $1,216 whereas someone under observation would be left to pay $10,368.36. Again, this does not reflect the doctor's fees for which both parties would be subject to pay 20% of cost. Therefore, this is likely an underestimate of the costs for inpatient care.

Medications Received in the Hospital

Medications administered to an inpatient are covered under Part A. Medications given to someone under observation are a whole other story. These medications are considered to be "self-administered drugs". It is a bit of a misnomer as most of these medications will not be administered by the patient himself but by nursing staff.

FINE PRINT:

Inpatient Medications

Covered by Medicare Part A

In fact, for reasons of safety, the hospital rarely lets you bring in your own medications. The hospital cannot know with certainty that those medications are what you claim they are. It is not an issue of paranoia but one of liability. If something were to happen to you while taking one of these medications, the hospital could be at risk for not having provided you appropriate medication. The hospital will usually provide you a medication in the same class if it does not have the specific one you take at home. If a medication does not have an alternative option available in the hospital pharmacy, the doctor may allow you to use your own medication if the medication is essential for your care. In order for someone to be able to use his own medications from home, the healthcare provider must write specific orders on the chart allowing this to happen.

The limited number of drugs that are covered under Medicare Part B will continue to be covered during an observation stay. Please refer to Chapter 4 for a more in-depth discussion. For medications not covered under Part B, you will receive a bill for the full charges from the healthcare facility.

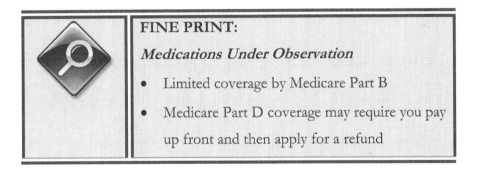

FINE PRINT:

Medications Under Observation

- Limited coverage by Medicare Part B
- Medicare Part D coverage may require you pay up front and then apply for a refund

If you have Medicare Part D for prescription coverage, these drugs could potentially be covered. Hospital formularies are limited and may not match what is covered by your Part D plan. Most often you will be charged the cost of the drugs by the hospital and will have to send a claim to your Part D plan to get reimbursed.

The Big Picture

If things stand as they do, inpatient admissions are in Medicare's crosshairs. CMS is allowing hospitals to get their feet wet with the new regulations, delaying potential fines for failure to comply with the 2-Midnight Rule until March 2015. Chart audits, however, are underway.

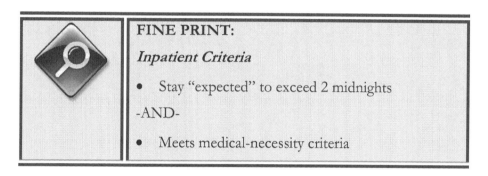

FINE PRINT:

Inpatient Criteria

- Stay "expected" to exceed 2 midnights

-AND-

- Meets medical-necessity criteria

There is a lot of confusion about what the rules mean. Some hospitals assume that after two midnights, all cases are inpatient appropriate. Taken to an extreme, that assumption almost implies that hospitals should keep their patients in the hospital longer just so they can attain inpatient status. There are so many things wrong with this. For one, this would add potentially unnecessary days of care to a hospital stay and with that added costs. It makes healthcare less efficient and also decreases availability of resources to those who may need a hospital bed. The 2-Midnight Rule was surely not intended to cost Medicare more money in the end. Medicare coverage requires both medical necessity and an "expected" time requirement that exceeds two midnights, though, like anything, there are exceptions to the rules.

You have a right to know whether you are being admitted as an inpatient or if you are being placed under observation. Ask your healthcare provider early on in the course of your hospital stay. You may not be able to sway the doctor to admit you one way or the other. They have to do their job and base their orders on medical necessity. The healthcare providers risk being audited by Medicare otherwise and

those audits could have consequences on their career. Your being aware of your inpatient vs. observation status is important as you should be involved in decisions on how much testing should be allowed under the circumstances. Costs may be a big factor for you to consider.

Ms. Jones Goes to the Hospital

Ms. Jones fractured her pelvic bone. She is unable to bear weight, requires IV medication for pain control and needs consultation with Physical Therapists to get her walking again. Her stay exceeds two midnights, but is a hospital stay medically necessary when she could be receiving Physical Therapy at home? What do you think?

Chapter 8 – Medicare in the Nursing Home and Beyond

After her pelvic fracture, Ms. Jones remained weak and frail. It was difficult to try to walk on her own, even with assistance. Her pain remained uncontrolled even with IV pain medication. Her doctor ordered a CT scan of the hip and found a fracture that had not been seen on the x-ray. She then had hip surgery. The Physical Therapist who took care of her in the hospital thought she was not strong enough to go home, at least not yet. Her doctor agreed. Ms. Jones needed extended care.

Ms. Jones could not stay in the hospital indefinitely. If you don't know the reason, you will learn it has more than a bit to do with dollars and cents. Medicare may not consider an extended hospital stay medically necessary. Those magic words again!

In particular, Medicare won't cover for custodial care. The phrase may seem a bit strange at first but it essentially means that Medicare does not want to babysit. If services can be performed somewhere other than a hospital where expenses are highest, then Medicare wants you to go to that somewhere else as soon as possible.

If Medicare does not consider her Physical Therapy medically necessary for hospital inpatient care, where does that put Ms. Jones? It puts her, hopefully, in a skilled nursing facility. The question is: does she qualify?

Skilled Nursing Facilities

A skilled nursing facility or SNF is exactly what it sounds like. It is a place where a person can be provided nursing care from people with qualified skills and medical expertise. Examples of skilled nursing facilities may include qualified nursing homes and rehabilitation centers. When you think about it, a hospital technically is also a skilled nursing facility. You stay in a facility where you receive nursing care and more. However, Medicare chooses to categorize hospitals in a different way. Hospitals are acute care facilities and are considered a higher level of care than a SNF.

Despite the distinction between a hospital and a SNF, Medicare Part A is the part of Medicare that provides coverage for both. We discussed the terms for hospital inpatient coverage in Chapter 7 but a whole new set of rules are put in place for care beyond those hospital walls.

Skilled Care

In order for Medicare to cover a SNF admission, it must first see that skilled care is required on a daily basis. That care must be ordered by a healthcare provider. For the purposes of Medicare, your care is considered daily even if the therapy services are offered only 5 or 6 days a week.

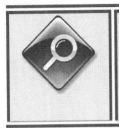

FINE PRINT:

Skilled services must be offered at least 5 days per week to meet criteria for a Medicare approved SNF stay.

To be considered skilled care, the services must be performed or supervised by trained professionals. In addition to physicians, physician assistants and advanced practice nurse practitioners, other qualifying professionals include audiologists, licensed practical nurses, occupational therapists, speech-language pathologists, physical therapists and registered nurses.

The skilled services covered by Medicare include the following:

- Occupational Therapy services
- Physical Therapy services
- Skilled nursing care
- Speech-Language Pathology services

Custodial care alone is not considered sufficient for Medicare coverage. For example, some patients may need assistance in bathing, dressing, toileting and managing colostomy bags or urinary catheters. Some may need help getting in and out of bed while others may need help in feeding and taking their medications or supplying their oxygen. All of these activities are important to the care of the patient but fall under custodial care. These services are offered in nursing homes but alone do not meet the level of acuity required for Medicare Part A coverage.

Other items covered by Medicare for those admitted to a SNF would include:

- Ambulance transportation to other healthcare facilities as medically necessary
- Dietary counseling
- Meals
- Medical supplies and equipment
- Medications
- Meals
- Semi-private room (you may have to share a room)
- Social service

SNF Timelines

Keeping all the different Medicare timelines straight can be quite a chore. There are timelines needed to qualify for SNF coverage, how long the coverage lasts and rules on when and if you can restart SNF care.

Medicare will not cover a stay in a SNF unless you are first admitted to a hospital as an inpatient. Chapter 7 showed us the complexities of the inpatient admission process. Transferring to a SNF after that hospital stay is even more complicated.

Not only must you be admitted as an inpatient but you must be admitted as an inpatient for three consecutive days in order to qualify for coverage. Further, the day you are discharged from the hospital does not count as one of the required three inpatient days. This means you must have been in the hospital for four days. Any days that you were placed under observation status do not count towards the requirement.

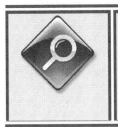

FINE PRINT:

SNF Admission Requirement

A minimum 3 day inpatient hospital stay (not including the day of discharge)

Once this criteria is met, there is a limited window on which you can be admitted into the SNF. Most people will be directly admitted to the SNF from the hospital but there may be situations where there is a delay in SNF care. Perhaps someone wants to see how well he or she does with home health services before committing to a SNF stay. To be covered by Medicare, you must be admitted to the SNF within 30 days of leaving the hospital.

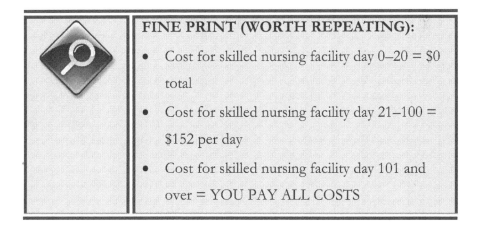

FINE PRINT (WORTH REPEATING):

- Cost for skilled nursing facility day 0–20 = $0 total
- Cost for skilled nursing facility day 21–100 = $152 per day
- Cost for skilled nursing facility day 101 and over = YOU PAY ALL COSTS

Medicare will cover the first 20 days of your SNF stay at no charge and days 21 to 100 at $152 per day. After that you are on your own. Medicare may cover costs for up to 100 days but your benefit window is only 60 days. This is where things get a bit more confusing.

FINE PRINT:

SNF benefits = 100 days

Benefit window = 60 days

Medicare may stop paying for SNF care for a number of reasons. You may leave a SNF because your condition is fully resolved. Once you are stable, you may choose to leave a SNF and pursue home health services instead. It could also be that while you are at a nursing home, skilled nursing care is stopped. That level of care may no longer be needed but custodial care may continue for your basic day to day living.

Life is never predictable. Your medical condition may deteriorate and you may again need skilled nursing care. This is when your benefit window comes into play. If you return to a SNF (any SNF, not necessarily the one where you originally stayed) within 30 days, Medicare will continue its coverage as if you never left the facility. Any remaining days from the original SNF 100 day coverage period will then be used.

If you return to the SNF between 31 and 59 days from your SNF stay, Medicare will require that you have a new three day inpatient hospital admission. Your current coverage window would continue. Any days already used would count toward the 100 days of coverage.

If you return to the SNF 60 days or later, again you will require a new three day inpatient hospital admission but you will start a new benefit and coverage period, starting with SNF day #0.

Non-Medicare Coverage for a SNF Stay

The sad truth is that Medicare offers little in the way of long-term care. Many people need nursing care as they age, whether that care falls into the skilled categories discussed previously or for basic everyday needs. Vision can become impaired. Balance issues creep in for some people. Cognitive decline can impact one's ability to be independent. Altogether, safety can be a serious concern as people age. According to the CDC, one out of three people over the age of 65 experiences a fall every year. There were 2.3 million injuries from falls in 2010 that resulted in 662,000 hospital stays.

FACT CHECK:

1 in 3 people over the age of 65 experience a fall every year

Long-term stays in a nursing home are not covered by Medicare. That leaves little in the way of options for care at one of these facilities to be covered. The costs of nursing home care can be staggering. In 2010, the average cost for a semi-private or shared room was $205 per day or $6,235 per month. That's $74,820 per year! A private room cost more at $229 per day, $6,965 per month, or $83,580 per year.

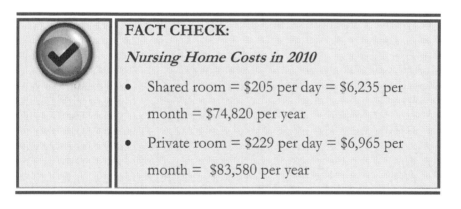

FACT CHECK:

Nursing Home Costs in 2010

- Shared room = $205 per day = $6,235 per month = $74,820 per year
- Private room = $229 per day = $6,965 per month = $83,580 per year

Some private insurance plans may offer coverage for nursing home stays through a managed care plan or long-term care insurance. For these private plans, a contract agreement between the insurance company and the specific nursing home is needed for you to be provided coverage. From my experience, you may be hard-pressed to find an insurance plan that covers enough of the needed services without being subject to an exorbitant monthly premium. Also, these plans are unlikely to cover the entire cost of the nursing home stay, which adds more monthly fees for you to pay.

A more common option for many people is to default to Medicaid. Medicaid offers healthcare services to Americans with low incomes. It is funded on federal and state levels but primarily managed by state governments. For this reason, eligibility for Medicaid will vary state by state. With resistance from certain states to implement certain provisions of the Affordable Care Act, Medicaid coverage remains a bit unpredictable at this time. This would be a whole book unto itself. Medicaid may allow for nursing home coverage at certified, i.e., government-approved, nursing homes.

For those who do not meet financial eligibility for Medicaid or have private insurance, they most likely will need to rely on their savings. Half of all nursing home care falls under this category. Once personal resources are depleted, those people may become eligible for Medicaid. Sadly, this is what I have witnessed more often than not.

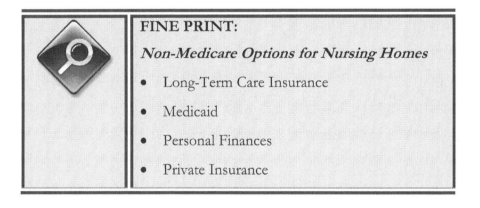

FINE PRINT:

Non-Medicare Options for Nursing Homes

- Long-Term Care Insurance
- Medicaid
- Personal Finances
- Private Insurance

Hospice Care

Long-term care at a nursing home is one thing but end-of-life care is another. Hospice is end-of-life care provided by qualified professionals to assist you and your family through a terminal illness.

These can be challenging times, both emotionally and physically, and a team of hospice-trained individuals will be available to ease your transition. This team may include physicians, nurse practitioners, nurses, counsellors, occupational therapists, physical therapists, speech-language pathologists, social workers, hospice aides and volunteers. A doctor who specializes in hospice care will be assigned to you but you may also receive care from your regular primary care provider. A hospice nurse and physician will be on-call for you 24 hours a day 7 days a week.

Once a physician certifies that an individual is terminally ill and expected to live less than 6 months, that individual becomes eligible for Hospice care. This is very important. Medicare requires that a physician make this certification, not any other type of licensed provider. After the initial certification is made, another healthcare provider, i.e., an advanced practice nurse practitioner or a physician assistant, may step in as the primary caregiver if preferred by the patient.

As we all know, doctors are not God. At best, the doctor can only use statistical estimates as a point of reference. We are all unique. These estimates may be too short or too long. What these life expectancies allow is for people to make their end-of-life plans if they so choose.

Some people become angry when a doctor tells them how much longer they may have to live. I can assure you no doctor likes to do it. It is an uncomfortable and often dreary discussion. The doctor is only trying to provide you information about the limited options to treat your condition. You, not the doctor, are the one who decides how to use that information. In the end, many people hope to prove the doctor wrong by living long past the deadline. Good for them! For the purposes of Hospice care, 6 months or less is the amount of time you are expected to live before Medicare will pay for services.

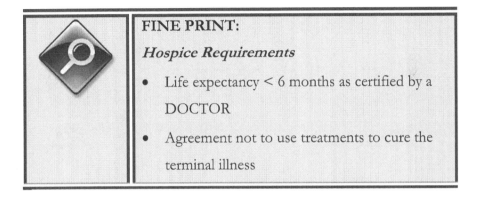

FINE PRINT:

Hospice Requirements

- Life expectancy < 6 months as certified by a DOCTOR
- Agreement not to use treatments to cure the terminal illness

Once a terminal diagnosis is made, Hospice care may be pursued if a decision is made to forego treatments that would attempt to cure the condition. For example, someone on Hospice would not be allowed to have chemotherapy to treat cancer if that cancer was the diagnosis that put him in Hospice in the first place. Chemotherapy would be an attempted treatment to cure the condition.

Your healthcare provider may have tried treatments that did not work or may find that the harms and side effects of other treatments may outweigh the benefits. Whatever the case may be, choosing Hospice care is a thoughtful decision to be made between the healthcare provider and his patient. Families are often involved in these complex decisions. I encourage family meetings with the provider to discuss the issues involved in making an informed choice.

Hospice care may be provided in your home or a Medicare-approved hospice facility, hospital hospice unit or nursing home.

What Hospice Does and Does Not Cover

Becoming a Hospice patient does not mean that all care is cut off. Palliative care, or comfort care, will allow symptom relief to ease any pain or suffering. Hospice provides an array of services to the patient including doctor services, dietary counseling, grief counseling, homemaker services, medical supplies and equipment, medications for comfort care, nursing care, Occupational Therapy, Physical Therapy, Social Work services and Speech-Language Pathology services.

Hospice may also allow for inpatient stays if needed for comfort care, i.e., pain and symptom control for the terminal condition. Respite care is a placement option that may offer relief for those caring for the patient in the home. Both of these are provided as short-term options only and must be approved and arranged by the Hospice team for Medicare to pay. Medicare covers respite services but requires a 5% copay.

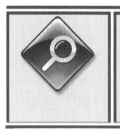

FINE PRINT:

Short-Term Hospice Services

Inpatient stays for pain or symptom control

Respite care

There may be times when a condition other than the terminal illness requires medical attention. For example, a urinary tract infection could cause unnecessary discomfort or even lead to complications with bacteria getting into the blood stream. Emergency room and even hospital care may be needed to treat and cure the condition. In this case, antibiotics would definitively treat the infection.

Original Medicare (Part A and Part B) may cover these services but it is best that you contact your hospice team before pursing treatment. The team will determine officially whether the condition is related to your terminal illness. You do not want to lose your Hospice benefits if you receive treatments that do not meet criteria.

Medicare, however, will not cover medications or treatments intended to cure your terminal condition. If new treatments become available or your condition changes, you may consider stopping Hospice care to pursue these options. Care from a provider not on or approved by your Hospice team will also not be covered.

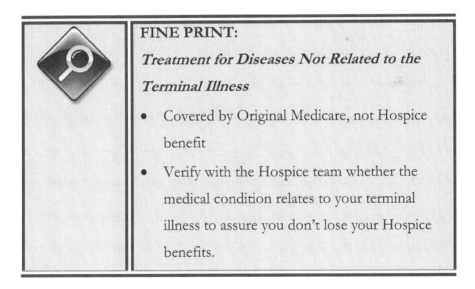

FINE PRINT:

Treatment for Diseases Not Related to the Terminal Illness

- Covered by Original Medicare, not Hospice benefit
- Verify with the Hospice team whether the medical condition relates to your terminal illness to assure you don't lose your Hospice benefits.

Logistics of Hospice

To be enrolled in Hospice, you must have both Medicare Part A and Part B benefits. The monthly premiums, deductibles, copays and coinsurance apply for Medicare-covered services as discussed in Chapter 3.

Hospice services are covered by Medicare Part A. The majority of Hospice services are covered with the following exceptions:

1. Room and board is not covered whether you are at home or in a Medicare-approved Hospice facility. This does not include inpatient hospital stays approved by the Hospice team.

2. Medications for pain and symptom control may require a copay up to $5 when you are at home. Medicare covers inpatient medications.

3. Respite care requires a 5% copay of the Medicare-approved amount.

Hospice is broken down into a series of benefit periods. The first two periods are at 90 day intervals. Subsequent benefit periods start every 60 days. A doctor must certify that you have a terminal illness at the start of each benefit period. As you can see, Hospice care can extend long after the initial expected 6 month interval. Again, doctors can't see into the future. They can only use statistics to give an estimate about someone's life expectancy. The 6 month life expectancy is what makes you initially eligibly for Hospice care in the first place.

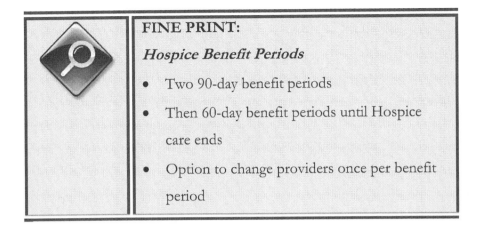

The benefit periods allow Medicare to confirm that you have a terminal illness and that coverage should continue. They also allow you an opportunity to change your healthcare providers if you want. You can only do this once during each benefit period.

Ms. Jones Needs Skilled Care

Ms. Jones was initially placed under observation after her fall. Once a hip fracture was discovered on the CT scan, her status was changed by her healthcare provider and she was admitted as in inpatient. She had hip surgery and stayed in the hospital for three consecutive days as an inpatient. This made her eligible for a SNF stay to continue Physical Therapy and Occupational Therapy services as part of her rehabilitation. Her stay will be covered free for the first 20 days and at $152 per day up to a total of 100 days.

She had a good recovery and was eager to return home. She was discharged from the SNF after 20 days and continued to receive Physical Therapy and Occupational Therapy as an outpatient, meaning she visited a facility two to three times per week for care. However, she had another fall and her condition worsened. She needed skilled nursing care again. Because she left the SNF only 2 weeks ago, she was still eligible to go back into the SNF without needing to go back to the hospital first. Medicare will charge her $152 per day since she would be considered to be on day 21 of her coverage benefit.

The rules can be tricky to navigate. By reading the fine print, you can understand how Medicare covers your needs for skilled care.

Chapter 9 – You and Medicare

"In the end it is not the years in your life that count. It is the life in your years."

— *Abraham Lincoln*

I hope you have found this book helpful to you. It addresses the most common questions I have had both patients and healthcare providers ask me about Medicare.

You will be surprised that after reading this book, you may actually know more about the Medicare program than many of the providers who care for you. In medical school, there has been limited training on the subject in recent years. For those doctors practicing for decades or longer, they may not have had any training at all. As Medicare evolves at a rapid pace, there is rarely someone actively reaching out to formally train medical providers on the changes. Your healthcare providers are doing the best they can to give you quality patient care. Adding the burden of administrative responsibilities has been a daunting task for some. Many of what they learn about Medicare is from simplified summaries and worksheets.

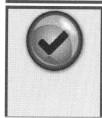
This is why you and your provider need to work together. The phrase patient-physician relationship is tossed around quite a bit. The way I see it, some relationships can be healthy and others toxic. I prefer to think of these essential dynamics as the patient-physician TEAM. Working together, you can maximize your health. Open communication is the key. You may have helpful information to share with your provider that can also help them care for other patients.

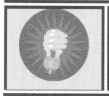
This chapter is a summary and rundown of key points throughout the book with some worksheets to help you on your way. The exact numbers used for calculations are based on 2014 data but will change annually.

MEDICARE ELIGIBILITY	Yes	No
#1 Are you a United States citizen or a legal U.S. resident for at least 5 years? **If no, stop here. You are not eligible for Medicare. If yes, continue on to see if you are eligible.**		
#2 Are you age 65 or older? **If yes, you are eligible for Medicare.**		
#3 Do you have kidney disease that requires dialysis or a kidney transplant AND one of the following: **1.** Eligibility for Social Security Disability Insurance (SSDI) or Railroad Retirement Board (RRB) **2.** At least 40 hours of Medicare-eligible employment by you, your spouse, or a guardian if you are a dependent. **If yes, you are eligible for Medicare.**		
#4 Do you have amyotrophic lateral sclerosis (ALS), also known as Lou Gehrig's disease, AND eligibility for SSDI or RRB? **If yes, you are eligible for Medicare.**		
#5 Have you been on disability with SSDI for more than 24 months? **If yes, you are eligible for Medicare.**		

MEDICARE ESSENTIALS	Answer Here		
Date you turned 65?			
Date you applied for Medicare?			
# months between the two dates = missed eligibility date*			
# years between the two dates = missed eligibility date*			
Did you work in Medicare-taxed employment?	Yes	No	
If yes, for how many quarters?	<30	31-39	40+
Does your provider accept Medicare for payment?	Yes	No	
Does your provider accept Medicare assignment? **	Yes	No	

*Missed eligibility dates apply to applicants who meet Medicare eligibility by age criteria. If you apply for Medicare more than 3 months after your 65th birthday, you missed your eligibility date.

** This is distinct from accepting Medicare for payment and is important because it decides how much your health provider can charge you for services. For definitions of any terms, please refer to Chapters 2 and 3.

Medicare Part A Costs Checklist

MEDICARE PART A	Answer Here
Monthly Premium *(Based on how many quarters you worked in Medicare taxed employment)* • For < 30 quarters = $234 • For 31–39 quarters = $426 • For 40+ quarters = Free	
Missed eligibility in years (MEY) *(If 1 year or more, please continue below)*	
How much you will pay extra per month: *Monthly Premium × 0.1*	
How long you will pay the late penalty: *MEY multiplied by 2*	_____ years

Medicare Part B Costs Checklist

MEDICARE PART B	Answer Here
Monthly Premium $104.90–$335.70 (see table in Chapter 3) *(Based on income tax from 2 years ago)*	
Deductible	$147 per year
Missed eligibility in years (MEY) *(If 1 year or more, please continue below)*	
How much you will pay extra per month *Monthly Premium x 0.1 x MEY*	
How long you will pay the late penalty	As long as you have Part B

Prescription Costs Checklist

MEDICARE PART D	Answer Here
Monthly Premium Minimum (National Base Beneficiary Premium) = $32.42 *(Based on specific plan you choose)*	
Deductible $0–$310 annually *(Based on specific plan you choose)*	
Additional Premium Costs $0–$69.30 (see table in Chapter 3) *(Based on income tax from 2 years ago)*	
Missed eligibility in months (MEM) *(If 3 months or more, please continue below)*	
How much you will pay extra per month *National Base Beneficiary Premium* $\times$ *0.01* $\times$ *MEM*	
How long you will pay the late penalty	As long as you have Part D (if you are over 65 years old).

The following table will help you to track your medication expenses as you approach and enter the Donut Hole. To use the table, fill in how much you spend into each field. Fill in the first column. Only after your expenses exceed $2,850 do you begin to fill in the second column.

	Pre-Donut Hole $0–$2,850	Donut Hole * $2,850–$4,550 ($1,750)
Monthly Premiums		Do not count
Part D Deductible		Do not count
Copays/ Coinsurance (PAID BY YOU)**		
January		
February		
March		
April		
May		
June		
July		
August		
September		
October		
November		
December		
Additional Rx Costs (PAID BY MEDICARE)***		
TOTAL:		

* Reminder that medications not covered by your Medicare Part D plan or medications purchased outside of the United States will not count towards your Donut Hole costs.

** Coinsurance during the Donut Hole is 47.5% of cost for brand-name medications and 72% of cost for genetic medications.

*** See Medicare expense sheet on the following page.

Medicare will provide you with a beneficiary notice for services rendered. Take those numbers relating to your Part D plan and enter them into the table. As noted in the previous table, enter information into the first column until total costs from both tables exceed $2,850. At that time, you may then begin to fill the Donut Hole column as needed.

Additional Rx Costs (PAID BY MEDICARE)	Pre-Donut Hole $0–$2,850	Donut Hole $2,850–$4,550 ($1,750)
January		
February		
March		
April		
May		
June		
July		
August		
September		
October		
November		
December		
TOTAL:		

These tables will allow you to monitor where you stand in regard to the Donut Hole.

Preventive Services Checklist for EVERYONE

Service	How Often Covered*	Date Done	Date Due
Alcohol Abuse Screening	Annually		
Blood Pressure Check	Annually		
Colon Cancer Screening: Barium Enema**	• Every 48 months • Every 24 months if high risk		
Colon Cancer Screening: Colonoscopy**	• Every 120 months • Every 48 months after a flexible sigmoidoscopy • Every 24 months if high risk		
Colon Cancer Screening: Fecal Occult Blood Test	Annually		
Colon cancer screening: Flexible Sigmoidoscopy**	• Every 48 months • Every 120 months after a screening colonoscopy		
Depression Screening	Annually		
Lipid Screening	Once every 5 years		
Vaccination: Flu Shot	Annually every flu season		
Vaccination: Pneumonia Shot	One time only		

*Only one timeline in the list is needed to qualify unless otherwise stated.

**You normally only pursue one of these tests at a time. If there is an abnormality detected on the test, one of the other listed tests may be pursued for further evaluation. It will likely be counted as a diagnostic as opposed to a preventive procedure. Different costs will apply.

Preventive Services Checklist for MEN

Service	How Often Covered	Date Done	Date Due
Digital Rectal Exam	Annually		
PSA Test	Annually		

Service	How Often Covered	Date Done	Date Due
Pap Smear	Every 24 months for all women Every 12 months for women with: • Abnormal Pap test within last 36 months • Childbearing age High risk for cervical or vaginal cancer		
Mammogram	Women 35–39 years old: • One baseline mammogram Women 40+ years old: • Every 12 months		

Preventive Services Checklist for THOSE WHO QUALIFY

Check off any criteria you meet in the **Conditions Needed to Qualify** column. Ask your provider whether you should pursue these preventive options. Only one condition is needed to qualify.

Service	Conditions Needed to Qualify*	How Often Covered
Aortic Aneurysm Screening	☐ Family history of aortic aneurysm ☐ Men 65–75 years old who smoked > 100 cigarettes	Once
Bone Density Study	☐ Estrogen deficiency/menopause ☐ Osteoporosis on drug therapy ☐ Prednisone or steroid drug use ☐ Primary hyperparathyroidism ☐ X-rays suggestive osteopenia, osteoporosis or vertebral fracture	Every 24 months
Counseling: Obesity	☐ BMI > 30	Annually
Counseling: Tobacco	☐ Current tobacco use	8 sessions over 12 months

Service	Conditions Needed to Qualify*	How Often Covered
Diabetes Screening	☐ BMI > 30 ☐ High blood pressure ☐ High cholesterol ☐ High sugars If you have 2 of the following: ☐ Age at least 65 years old ☐ Birth of a child weighing > 9 pounds ☐ BMI 25–30 ☐ Family history for diabetes ☐ Gestational diabetes	Annually
Diabetes Training	☐ Diabetes	Annually • Up to 10 hours the 1st year • Up to 2 hours 2nd year onward
Medical Nutrition Therapy	☐ Diabetes ☐ Kidney disease ☐ Kidney transplant within last 36 months	Annually

Service	Conditions Needed to Qualify*	How Often Covered
Hepatitis B Vaccine	☐ Diabetes ☐ End stage renal disease ☐ Healthcare workers ☐ Hemophilia ☐ Past blood transfusions	One vaccination series
Hepatitis C Screening	☐ Born between 1945 and 1965 ☐ History of blood transfusion before 1992 ☐ History of injected illicit drug use	• One-time screening for everyone • Additional annual screening for those who continue to use injectable illicit drugs
HIV Screening	☐ "At high risk" ☐ Pregnant ☐ You request the test	• Annually • Multiple times during pregnancy
Sexually Treated Infection Screening and/or Counseling	☐ "At high risk"	Annually

Hospital Costs Checklist

HOSPITAL STAY	Costs	
Are you placed Under Observation? If yes, please stop here. *You will be billed for services under Medicare Part B.*	Yes	No
Are you admitted as an Inpatient? If yes, please continue. *Medicare Part A will pay for hospital services.* *Medicare Part B will pay for doctor services.*	Yes	No
Total # Days as an Inpatient (TD-IP)		
How much you will pay for the first 60 days: $1,216 deductible total, add amount to cost column.		
How much you will pay for days 61–90 (30 days): Calculation: # days x $304 per day		
How much you will pay for days 90 and over: Calculation: # days x $608 per day		

Skilled Nursing Facility Costs Checklist

SKILLED NURSING FACILITY STAY*	Costs
Total # Days in the SNF (TD-SNF)	
How much you will pay for days 0–20: $0 total	
How much you will pay for days 21–100: Calculation: # days x $152 per day	

* You are eligible for a Medicare-covered SNF stay if you were admitted for three consecutive Inpatient days in a row, NOT including the day you were discharged from the hospital.

Ms. Jones Understands Medicare

Ms. Jones has been on a full journey. Her journey has brought her from the home to the hospital to a skilled nursing facility. She understands the breakdown of Medicare and what it does and does not cover. She also understands how much it will cover and how much is left for her to pay out of pocket. In this climate of healthcare reform, there are likely more changes to come.

References

"Change is the law of life. And those who look only to the past or present are certain to miss the future."

— *John F. Kennedy*

Medicine is in a state of flux. The Affordable Care Act has made significant changes that affect our country's views on what constitutes quality healthcare. While the law has not changed someone's eligibility for Medicare, it has impacted Medicare's services as discussed throughout the course of this book. Other changes are sure to follow under future administrations.

Understanding your options is key to navigating the healthcare marketplace.

Diagnosis Life, LLC

I founded **Diagnosis Life** in 2010 as a way to educate the public about common health issues. Since that time, my passion for making a difference in healthcare has only grown. My clinical and administrative experience puts me in a position to offer a unique brand of expertise. I hope that the information presented here shines light on concerns you may have had about Medicare. Simplifying the terms and FINE PRINT makes it easier to understand how to medically and cost-effectively navigate Medicare. You deserve to get the most out of the Medicare experience for the least cost.

To connect with **Diagnosis Life**, please visit one of the following sites:

Web Site: www.diagnosislife.com

Facebook: www.facebook.com/diagnosislife

You can reach me through either site listed above. Please direct messages to me through the CONTACT field on the web site. I can be made available for speaking engagements or individual consultations.

I will not, however, provide direct medical advice at this time. In my experience, a medical condition does require hands-on evaluation. I encourage you to seek any medical care with your current or local healthcare provider at your earliest convenience.

Recommended Web Sites

Many online resources are available to you. Be sure to use sites that have reliable source material. Professional organizations, companies and government web sites will be more detail oriented. Personal web sites may be too subjective to guide you on the right path. You should be wary of them unless they can verify their credentials.

Below are web sites I referred to frequently as I researched this book. You will find sound information here to add to what you have read in these pages.

Medicare.gov (Official U.S. government Medicare web site):

www.medicare.gov

The Centers for Disease Control and Prevention (CDC):

www.cdc.gov

Healthcare Bluebook (owned by CAREOperative, LLC):

www.healthcarebluebook.com

Medicare.com (Non-government web site privately owned and operated by eHealthInsurance Services, Inc.):

www.medicare.com

Made in the USA
Charleston, SC
22 August 2014